Probably Someday Cancer

Genetic Risk and Preventative Mastectomy

Kim Horner

Foreword by Sue Friedman

Number 9 in the Mayborn Literary Nonfiction Series

U**N**T
PRESS

University of North Texas Press
Mayborn Graduate Institute of Journalism
Denton, Texas

10 9 8 7 6 5 4 3 2 1

Permissions:
University of North Texas Press
1155 Union Circle #311336
Denton, TX 76203-5017

The paper used in this book meets the minimum requirements of the American National Standard for Permanence of Paper for Printed Library Materials, z39.48.1984. Binding materials have been chosen for durability.

Library of Congress Cataloging-in-Publication Data

Names: Horner, Kim, 1967- author.
Title: Probably someday cancer : genetic risk and preventative mastectomy / by Kim Horner ; foreword by Sue Friedman.
Other titles: Mayborn literary nonfiction series ; no. 9.
Description: Denton, Texas : University of North Texas Press, Mayborn Graduate Institute of Journalism, [2019] | Series: Number 9 in the Mayborn literary nonfiction series
Identifiers: LCCN 2018047763| ISBN 9781574417517 (cloth : alk. paper) | ISBN
   9781574417579 (ebook)
Subjects: LCSH: BRCA genes. | Breast--Cancer--Genetic aspects. | Horner, Kim, 1967- | Breast--Surgery--Patients--Biography. | Breast--Cancer--Prevention. | Mastectomy. | LCGFT: Autobiographies.
Classification: LCC RC268.44.B73 H66 2019 | DDC 616.99/449--dc23
LC record available at /https://lccn.loc.gov/2018047763

Probably Someday Cancer: Genetic Risk and Preventative Mastectomy is Number 9 in the Mayborn Literary Nonfiction Series

The electronic edition of this book was made possible by the support of the Vick Family Foundation.

For Margaret, Lucy Belle,
mom and all women and men facing hereditary risk
of breast and ovarian cancer.

Contents

Forword

by Sue Friedman

For anyone who is concerned with hereditary cancer, making decisions about genetic counseling, testing and treatment can be frustratingly complex. Many questions arise, and the answers aren't always as simple and as straightforward as we might expect or like them to be. It's good news that more and more resources are available to individuals who are seeking answers about their hereditary status and potential risk for cancers. It's not-so-good news that some of those resources are better than others, muddying the quest to answer the question: "Should I, or shouldn't I?" But how do you know the difference?

From the title to its final words, *Probably Someday Cancer* speaks to the ambiguous, confusing status of being diagnosed with a BRCA mutation and facing increased cancer risk. With the ease and comfort of a trusted friend, Kim Horner expertly takes you through her personal journey, sharing her thoughts and evolution around the difficult decisions that she had to make about genetic counseling, testing and risk management. This is a moving and candid memoir, but it is also much more than that. In *Probably Someday Cancer* Kim adeptly uses her frustrations, her experiences and her education to help readers find their way through the hereditary cancer journey. She shares the resources, research, conversations and considerations that contributed to her decision making, including some lesser covered topics, such as how legal protections and financial considerations can impact medical care. *Probably Someday Cancer* provides an up-to-date, timely guide for anyone who has wondered, "Am I at elevated risk for cancer?" For those who have learned that they are at high risk, the book helps answer the question, "What should I do next?"

Among those of us who have received a serious medical diagnosis and have had to navigate complex medical decisions, who hasn't felt marginalized and isolated? Yet who among us can forget the wondrous feeling of the first time we reached out to other people, either in person or online, and learned that we are not alone? This book captures that feeling so well and provides so much more. Ms. Horner's journalistic skills and insights enrich her book and its message. It's obvious that she has done her homework, as she provides context and balance to the aspects of genetic testing and risk reduction, especially those that foster controversy. The informative text is infused with her personal story and insights that guided her decision-making process. *Probably Someday Cancer* is the book that I wish I had when I was diagnosed with a BRCA2 mutation and faced challenging decisions in 1997 at the age of 35.

Retail shelves are lined with books about the cancer experience, including many that focus exclusively on the hereditary cancer experience. *Probably Someday Cancer* is a shining star in that collection; a book of unique insight and information told clearly and compassionately. It is sure to be a valuable addition to the library of every high-risk patient and family, and every provider who cares for them.

—Sue Friedman, DVM, Founder and Executive Director
of Facing Our Risk of Cancer Empowered (FORCE).

Introduction

When I was 41, I tested positive for a harmful BRCA2 mutation—an inherited genetic abnormality that gave me a scary high risk of developing breast cancer someday. The odds were so great, my doctor urged me to consider having an elective double mastectomy.

I was the same age at the time as my grandmother was when she died of breast cancer, leaving her three devastated children. My son was only a year old. The thought of anything happening to me was terrifying.

I didn't know anything about BRCA mutations when I got my test result in January 2009. It was more than four years before Angelina Jolie wrote in *The New York Times*[1] about her BRCA1 mutation and decision to have a risk-reducing double mastectomy. Jolie's article led many women to wonder if they, too, were at high risk; however, thankfully BRCA mutations are not common. About one in 400 people in the general population carry a harmful BRCA mutation, although the number rises to one in 40 among people of Ashkenazi Jewish heritage.[2] Breast cancers caused by BRCA mutations account for 5 to 10 percent of all breast cancers.[3]

For those of us with BRCA mutations, what do you do with a diagnosis that you *probably* will get cancer someday? It could be in a year. It could be decades away. On the other hand, you may never get sick. The ability to uncover the medical information encoded in our genes gives us a chance to prevent some diseases or at least try to catch them early. But it also can force what feel like impossible choices.

On one end, there's close screenings with alternating mammograms, MRIs and clinical breast exams to try to catch any cancer early. On the other, there's an elective surgery few would otherwise choose: a double mastectomy, or prophylactic bilateral mastectomy, to reduce the risk of breast cancer to less than 10 percent.[4] The right path was far from obvious. My doctors presented both strategies as rational choices, although my oncologist suggested I also take tamoxifen to lower my breast cancer risk if I did not have surgery. The National Comprehensive Cancer Network guidelines, which dictate the standard of care for high-risk patients, recommend that women with BRCA mutations receive enhanced screenings and consider preventative mastectomies. Most of my doctors would not advocate for or against the surgery. Instead, it would come down to what they called a "personal decision," one I felt completely unqualified to make given the stakes.

More and more of us may face these kinds of medical decisions now that genetic testing has become more affordable and available and we learn about other genetic risks for breast cancer and a growing list of diseases. My hope is that *Probably Someday Cancer* will help women and men with a hereditary risk of breast and ovarian cancer, their loved ones and anyone confronted with difficult medical decisions face their risk, take control of their healthcare, make informed decisions and feel less alone.

This book was written from a patient's perspective. I am not a medical expert, just a person who has spent countless hours researching BRCA mutations and consulting with physicians at numerous appointments over the years. *Probably Someday*

Cancer is intended to be a story of my experiences and how and why I came to my decisions rather than an authoritative source on BRCA mutations. Pinning down certain facts about BRCA mutations can be a challenge. For example, separate studies give different estimates about breast cancer risk for people with BRCA2 mutations. My 2009 test result from Myriad Genetic Laboratories, Inc. said that I had "as much as an 84 percent" risk of breast cancer by age 70, citing 1998 research in the *American Journal of Human Genetics*.[5] A 2007 study put the risk at 49 percent.[6] A large 2017 study in the *Journal of the American Medical Association* estimated that my risk was 69 percent by age 80.[7] An Internet search on the risk of breast cancer for women with a BRCA2 mutation will reveal a range of answers between those highs and lows. The bottom line is, there's no way, at least not yet, to know your exact risk on an individual level. In Chapter 1, I share the number in my lab report when I was diagnosed with a BRCA mutation because it is part of my story and it factored into my decision-making; however, it is not meant to be taken as the current estimated risk. I write more about the difficulty of knowing your exact risk in Chapter 2.

The information in this book comes from my experiences, interviews, medical journal articles and organizations that provide information including the National Cancer Institute and nonprofit organizations such as Facing Our Risk of Cancer Empowered (FORCE), Susan G. Komen and the American Cancer Society. I have sought guidance from medical experts to ensure that the information is accurate. I am grateful for the compassionate, excellent medical professionals: the breast surgeons, oncologists, gynecological oncologists, genetic counselors, gastroenterologists, nurse practitioners, nurses, radiologists, techs, admitting staff and so many others that I have met since I was diagnosed with a BRCA2 mutation. I have changed their names in this book to protect the privacy of the patient/ medical provider relationship. Conversations have been recreated by memory, my journals and notes. Details about appointments, diagnoses and medical information come from my medical records.

CHAPTER 1

Welcome to BRCAland

"I think that it brings power. . . . it brings actual evidence of something that is concrete, that is wrong, that is nobody's fault, with the awareness that there are things that can be done about it. Not simple, pretty things, but there is action that can be taken. And it saves lives."[1]

—Dr. Mary-Claire King, geneticist who pinpointed a genetic link to breast cancer in a region of chromosome 17, which she called BRCA1

(February 2009)

I don't have cancer. But here I am, sitting in a packed waiting room, waiting to see an oncologist. My doctor sent me here because last month, I found out that I have a harmful BRCA2 genetic mutation, an inherited genetic abnormality that puts me at a crazy high risk for breast and ovarian cancer. My lab result states that I have an "as much as an 84 percent risk of breast cancer," though I've seen other information that puts my risk at closer to 50 percent.[2]

The test result set off a flurry of appointments. Genetic counselor. Breast surgeon. Oncologist. Gynecological oncologist. MRI. The MRI, an extra layer of screening for high-risk patients, identified a "suspicious area." So, now I need a biopsy. Suddenly, I had a team of doctors with serious specialties who acted as if I was already sick.

The waiting room looks like any other. A couple rows of your basic wood chairs with mauve cushions, arranged close together. The oncology practice has a cold feel. No one is smiling. Maybe I'm in denial. Or it hasn't sunk in. I keep thinking I don't belong here. I'm 41—a lot younger than any of the patients surrounding me. I'm the same age that my grandmother, Lucy Belle, whom I never got to meet, was when she died of breast cancer. She never got to see her three children finish growing up. I think about my son, Leo. He's only a year old, still in diapers. I get occasional flashes of panic worrying about whether a tumor might be growing inside me right now. I don't look or feel sick. I feel fine, except for the queasy feeling in my stomach. I haven't lost my hair. A fragile-looking older woman across the room is wearing a pretty, light blue floral scarf over her bald head. A woman with gray stubbles of hair on her head sits next to her husband, both staring grimly at the floor. I didn't think of asking my husband or anyone else to come with me. After all, I'm not sick. Somehow going alone keeps it from feeling like a Big Deal. I wonder how much longer I will have to wait. I just want to get out of this place.

The waiting area is so quiet. People talk in library voices. Everything seems to be in slow motion. A nurse calls a man who appears to be in his 70s and leads him through a door next to a sign that says, "Infusion Room." No one hurries into a place like that. Magazines spread out on the table feature upbeat stories with photos of smiling cancer survivors. In one, a woman had lived several years with metastatic breast cancer, meaning the cancer had spread from the breast to other parts of her body. She was determined to see her young children graduate from college. The odds did not seem good. Not that the magazine's readers need to be reminded. There's a brochure filled with young, attractive, smiling, women who don't look like cancer patients modeling cute brightly colored scarves, hats and nicely coiffed wigs for women who lose their hair from chemotherapy. I get uncomfortable as I look at bras with pockets for foam or silicone "breast forms." Will I need one someday? As soon as that thought crosses my mind, my brain interrupts and I skip to my assignment at work and worry about whether I will get back in time to finish it.

The oncology office is busy despite the silence. I think of a sick twist on an old *Saturday Night Live* skit and the line goes through my head that cancer has been very, very good to this place. I feel like I'm on an assembly line. First the check-in counter, then the windowless waiting room. Then they call me into a station where I wait again, in one of four chairs facing a curtained-off area, this time to have blood drawn. It's next to the infusion room. I catch a glimpse of people in light blue chairs that recline, hooked up to tubes that deliver harsh chemicals that hopefully will shrink their tumors and save their lives, not without dragging them through the lowest rungs of hell first. I've never been inside an oncology practice. I feel ill just being there.

My doctor says I probably will get breast cancer someday. He sent me to the oncologist to find out what I can do to keep that from happening. I don't even know exactly what my risk is because there is such a range of estimates. Knowing you have a family history of cancer is one thing. Finding out your risk could be 50 percent or higher is something else. The average woman's risk is 12 percent, which is still too much.

I zone out and look at the carpet. A nurse calls my name. She takes me to an examination room. Weight. Blood Pressure. Temperature. Undress from the waist up. Gown open to front. Then it's time to sit, waiting, again. I scan email on my phone. A few minutes later, there's a light knock on the door. Dr. B comes in. She's a thin, petite woman around 60 in heels and a perfectly pressed white lab coat over a dress. She smiles. She seems nice. I sit in a chair while she types answers about my family history into her computer. Then she asks me to lie on the exam table for a clinical breast exam. It's my second in the past couple weeks. I'd had clinical breast exams by gynecologists who gently pressed into my breasts. Not these breast surgeons and oncologists. They push and dig to find any possible lump until you feel pulverized. Thankfully it's over within a couple of minutes.

Afterward, Dr. B says I can get dressed and she leaves the room. A few minutes later, I hear a tap on the door. She comes in, sits on a round rolling stool and types something into her computer. She mentions my upcoming biopsy.

"If we find anything, the breasts are going to have to come off," she says in a matter-of-fact way as if we were talking about having to replace my car tires.

Breasts . . . "come off?" That did it. The tears poured down my face.

Dr. B looked concerned and came closer. She put an arm lightly on my shoulder.

"Where is this coming from?" she said. Dr. B undoubtedly has given a lot of nightmare news to patients. On the scale of the news she has to deliver, this was barely a Category 1. But still.

I can't say anything. What is there to say? *Hmmmmm. I don't know. Maybe from the thought of my breasts having to "come off?"*

Everyone has two sets of BRCA1 and BRCA2 genes, one from each parent, that produce proteins that help repair damaged DNA, according to the National Cancer Institute (NCI), the federal government agency for cancer research and training.[3]

When the genes are working properly, they help suppress tumors. One of my BRCA2 genes, however, is broken. In addition to putting me at high risk for breast cancer, a BRCA2 mutation gives me an 11 percent to 17 percent risk of ovarian cancer. (Again, there is a range of estimates; it depends which study you look at.) This risk is more than 10 times higher than the risk of the average woman, according to the NCI.[4] (The risk is even higher for women with BRCA1 mutations: an estimated 39 percent of women who inherit a harmful BRCA1 mutation will develop ovarian cancer by age 70.)[5]

Breast and ovarian cancers associated with BRCA1 and BRCA2 mutations tend to strike at younger ages than non-BRCA related breast and ovarian cancers.[6] BRCA mutations raise the risk of breast cancer in men, although the threat is still low.[7] BRCA1 and BRCA2 mutations also have been linked to higher risks for other types of cancer, including pancreatic cancer.[8]

Of course, I may never get any of these cancers. There's no way to know. I'm not even sure how scared I should be.

Before the BRCA test, I was cautious but didn't worry too much about breast cancer. Now, I can't think about much else. I keep thinking about the fact that my grandmother died at the same age I am now. Her life ended at an age when mine feels like it is beginning. I've only been married a couple of years. I had my son, Leo, at 39 and work at a job I love, writing about issues like housing, homelessness and poverty at *The Dallas Morning News*. Sometimes my heart pounds so hard it feels like it could break open and I get flushed and shaky as I wonder if cancer is already growing inside me.

Because of our family history, I started getting annual mammograms when I was about 30. I always felt comfortable that if I developed cancer, the screenings would catch it early. My first scare came in my early 30s when my gynecologist became concerned about a lump in my left breast. I had a biopsy and thankfully, there was no cancer, although the pathology revealed that I had atypical ductal hyperplasia (ADH), an abnormal cell growth that put me at higher risk for breast cancer, according to the American Cancer Society.[9] At the time, in 2003, my doctors never suggested that I do anything about my risk beyond getting annual mammograms. My doctor had estimated my risk at about 18 percent using a common breast cancer risk assessment tool. My grandmother and great-grandmother died of breast cancer in their 40s, but my mom is in her 60s and has never had cancer. Her good fortune gave us a false sense of security. We had no idea, until the BRCA test, how deeply our breast cancer risk was stitched into our DNA.

I probably still wouldn't know if I didn't happen to fill out a voluntary questionnaire to assess my breast cancer risk when I went in for my annual mammogram. I answered a series of questions on a small tablet.

Do you have a family history of breast cancer?
Yes.
Have you had atypical ductal hyperplasia?
Yes. (Found in the biopsy when I was in my 30s.)
And then there was the family tree.
Grandmother Lucy. Diagnosed at 38. Died at 41.
Great-grandmother Margaret. Diagnosed at 39. Died at 45.
Great-aunt Katherine. Diagnosed with what we'd been told was a stomach cancer. Died in her 70s.

I turned in the tablet, got my mammogram and didn't think much more about it.

A week or so later, I got a letter:

"Based on the information you provided in the survey you do exhibit enough of these criteria to be at a higher than average risk of developing breast cancer. It is recommended that you contact your primary care provider or the Breast Cancer Risk Assessment Service to discuss options which are appropriate to your individual risk."

I called the number provided. Could I come in to meet with a nurse practitioner to discuss the assessment? Sure. I scheduled an appointment, maintaining a "why not?" attitude. I wasn't too worried.

I met with Donna, a nurse practitioner. She was concerned about the fact that I had been diagnosed with atypical ductal hyperplasia and that my grandmother and great-grandmother died in their 40s of breast cancer. She went over my family history.

Before the appointment, my mom said to make sure to tell her that I had a great-uncle who died of breast cancer. Her mother's brother. I had forgotten about that. It was a while back and I'd never met him.

When I told Donna, her eyes nearly popped out.

"You have a male in your family who died of breast cancer?"

"Yes, my grandmother's brother."

A male with breast cancer. A great-grandmother and grand-mother who died of breast cancer in their 40s. Atypical ductal hyperplasia. She said those were strong signs that our family may have a genetic mutation.

Donna asked if it was possible my great-great aunt had ovarian cancer rather than stomach cancer?

Huh? I had no idea.

"Sometimes women who were said to have died of stom-ach cancer actually had ovarian or uterine cancer," Donna said. "People didn't talk about those types of cancers back then."

What had been a fuzzy picture was coming into focus. If it was true—if my great-great aunt died of ovarian or uterine cancers—cancer may not be as limited and random in my family as I thought.

Donna suggested I meet with a genetic counselor, a specialist in genetics and counseling who helps people assess their risks and get tested for the BRCA mutation. The test, called BRACAnalysis, would be expensive, about $3,400, at the time. Insurance may or may not pay for it. The results might explain the devastation that cancer had caused in our family. She gave me a brochure from Myriad Genetic Laboratories Inc., a Salt Lake City, Utah, company that provides the test, that said "Be Ready Against Cancer." It said: "Even if there's a pattern of breast and/or ovarian cancer in your family, *cancer doesn't have to be inevitable.*"

I don't know what I had expected from the meeting, but it wasn't this. I thought that she would have me answer more questions and tell me my risk was around 18 percent like my doctor had said. I told her I needed to think about the testing. I already knew I had a family history. How would it help to know if it was caused by a BRCA mutation?

"Your insurance would pay for extra screenings, so you can catch any cancer early," Donna said. "And you could make decisions about your health."

What about the downsides of getting the BRCA test? Would I be labeled as a high-risk? Would it be a pre-existing condition that could allow insurers to deny coverage? Would I be able to get new insurance if I left my job? (This was before federal regulations in the Affordable Care Act made that illegal.) Could an employer fire me if they found out? Would my insurance pay for the test? (It did. I was fortunate. It's too expensive for some. Later, the Affordable Care Act mandated coverage for high-risk patients, but many women still struggle to pay for tests and screenings involved.)

It was a lot to take in. Of course, I found plenty of information on the Internet to fuel my fears and generate more questions. There was a new federal law at the time, the Genetic Information Nondiscrimination Act of 2008 (GINA), which protects people from discrimination based on genetics. Would it work in reality? I couldn't find any examples of people being denied health insurance based on their genetic predisposition to a disease. People on the message boards I searched complained about getting turned down for life insurance policies due to their BRCA mutation. Life insurance is important if you die. I wanted to live. I talked it over with my husband, my mom, my sisters. The topic was so new to all of us. I needed to learn more about BRCA and what a positive result would mean. Christmas was coming. I put it off. I didn't want to find out I had a mutation during the holidays.

After New Year's, I made the appointment with the genetic counselor. I didn't want to let fear keep me from being tested. I wanted to know. I hoped the test would rule out a BRCA mutation. After all, the mutations are not common, at least in the general population. I wasn't aware of my family having any Ashkenazi Jewish heritage. What were the chances I'd test positive?

At the appointment, the genetic counselor, Beth, took a blood sample to ship to Myriad, the only lab that provided the test at the time due to a patent. (The U.S. Supreme Court later ruled against that patent, opening the door for other companies to conduct the test.) With insurance, my portion thankfully was around $340, which was a lot of money but better than $3,400. After the appointment, I headed back to work. For the next several days, I tried not to think about the fact that more than a thousand miles away, someone might be analyzing my DNA.

A week later, Beth called to tell me my results were back. My heart pounded.

"Can you tell me the results over the phone?" I asked.

"No, we don't give results over the phone."

She asked if I could come the next day. Or I could come in that afternoon. This sounded bad. I was getting nervous. I told my boss I had to go to an appointment. I sped from *The News* downtown to Central Expressway to the hospital to meet the genetic counselor and tried to focus on the road rather than the tornado in my stomach.

I sat in the genetic counselor's tiny office. She pulled out a stack of papers. I could see the words "deleterious mutation." I had no idea what that meant. I thought it might be good news. I felt a moment of relief.

Until I saw Beth's face. She said I had the BRCA2 mutation.

"The results of this analysis are consistent with the germline BRCA2 mutation 8803delC, resulting in a premature truncation of the BRCA2 protein at amino acid position 2862. Although the exact risk of breast and ovarian cancer conferred by this specific mutation has not been determined, studies of this type of mutation in high-risk families indicate that deleterious mutations in BRCA2 may confer as much as an 84 percent risk of breast cancer and a 27 percent risk of ovarian cancer by age 70 in women (Am. J. Hum. Genet. 62:676–689, 1998). Mutations in BRCA2 have been reported to confer a 12 percent risk of a second breast cancer within five years of the first (J. Clin Oncol 17:3396–3402, 1998), as well as a 16 percent risk of subsequent ovarian cancer (J Natl Cancer Inst 91:1310–1315, 1999) . . ."

It turns out a deleterious mutation, as defined by the National Cancer Institute, is "a genetic alteration that increases an individual's susceptibility or predisposition to a certain disease or disorder. When such a variant (or mutation) is inherited, development of symptoms is more likely, but not certain. Also called disease-causing mutation, pathogenic variant, predisposing mutation, and susceptibility gene."[10]

I was stunned.

I had a mutation. The word itself even sounded awful, like *I* was a mutant.

This meant my grandmother and great-grandmother's cancers weren't just a couple cases of bad luck. It meant that their cancers probably were linked to my three great-great aunts' vague "stomach" cancers. It was much worse than I imagined. All these family cancers could be explained by this one error in our genetic code rather than random bad luck. None of these relatives had stood a chance against this mutation lurking in our genes.

We had caught a serial killer.

Questions and worries flooded my mind. *Is this really happening? I thought this test would rule out this BRCA thing. Will I get breast and/or ovarian cancer? Do I have it already? The area where my ovaries are hurts. Am I going to die from these cancers? If I have the BRCA2 mutation, my mom does too. My sisters could have it. My nephews could have it. My cousins could have it. My son could have it. What am I going to do? This is awful. Why did I do this test? What time is it? I need to get out of here. I should get back to work.*

"Do you have any sisters?" Beth asked.

"Yes, two."

"Your mom and sisters should get tested."

Since my test identified the exact location of the mutation in our DNA, my family members could get a simpler and less costly test. Beth gave me a sample letter to share with relatives—in my case uncles and cousins. It would be weird to get a letter like that out of the blue. One website recommended talking to relatives about BRCA before sending it.

Beth gave me a fact sheet that put my risk at between 56 to 87 percent. It was frustrating to get such a wide range. Which one was it? I might make different decisions based on the answer. Could this stuff be blown out of proportion? Could my real risk be even lower?

Problem is, nobody can tell you your individual risk. The commonly cited risk percentages come from a handful of studies based on various small populations. Some experts say that looking within your own family history can help fill in the picture. But that can be difficult, especially when some women in a family may have had vague cancers that nobody talked about.

The next step was to see Dr. A, a breast surgeon who worked in the same office as Donna.

I sat on the thin sheet of white paper that covered the hard vinyl examination table, wearing a light blue paper gown that opened in the front, trying to work out the lead to my story that day as I waited. The only sound was the crinkle of the paper when I fidgeted. I heard hushed voices outside the door. After a quick knock on the door, Dr. A and a nurse stepped in the room. Dr. A was tall with a big, friendly presence. Every day, he probably saw women who have cancerous tumors growing in their breasts. I was tumor-free, at least as far as we knew. My recent mammogram was clear. I didn't feel any lumps. Part of me still wondered why I was there.

Dr. A smiled, held out his hand and introduced himself. He was nice. He flipped through my chart. He looked up. He had a grave expression that scared me.

"Donna told me about your test results. I'm so sorry," he said. Dr. A looked down and talked as if I did have cancer. He looked so serious. I was surprised. I thought of saying, 'But I don't have cancer, you see.'

I opened the gown and sat bare-chested on the examination table, feeling awkward as Dr. A studied my chest. I was self-conscious about my breasts. They were small. A-cup. Dallas was one of the breast implant capitals of the United States, probably the world, where it's not unheard of for young women to get implants for their 18th birthday. I grew up seeing billboards advertise plastic surgery. Big boobs are definitely a big thing here. And if you don't have them, the message is that you're literally not measuring up. (As I got older, I increasingly realized that a smaller cup size has its benefits: I can only think of one time I caught a man besides a doctor staring at my breasts.)

"You'd be a good candidate for nipple-sparing mastectomies," he said, looking at my chest.

I must have had a blank look. I had no idea what he was talking about. And I wasn't sure I wanted to know.

"That's where you can keep your nipples," he said.

Oh. What a comfort. All this talk about mastectomies and whether I could keep my nipples was freaking me out.

"I can't get my head around the idea of surgery," I said.

"It would reduce your chance of getting cancer by 90 percent," Dr. A said. "Your risk would be lower than the average woman's risk."

Dr. A ordered an MRI. He said the MRI would provide a baseline. I'd get a mammogram once a year, followed by an MRI six months later. I'd be watched closely until I make up my mind about whether to have a double mastectomy, he said.

"What do *you* recommend for patients with BRCA mutations?" I asked.

"It's a personal decision," he said. "There's no right or wrong answer."

"I have no idea what to do," I said. My eyes started tearing up as I tried to dam a flood of fear, sadness and frustration about what to do.

"The BRCA test . . . it's a real Pandora's box," Dr. A said. "As we keep finding out more and more about genetic links to diseases, more and more people are going to face these types of difficult choices. It's a hard decision, maybe the hardest of any my patients face."

Even so, I knew that most of his patients would probably love to have that choice.

In Greek mythology, Pandora was given a box of evils including diseases, worries, crime and pain. Against orders not to open the box, her curiosity got the best of her and she released them into the world. She couldn't put them back in the box any more than I could undo my BRCA test. They say knowledge is power. I don't feel empowered. I feel like I have no control.

So, what do you do about a probably someday cancer? You don't know *if* it'll ever even strike. And you certainly don't know when. People diagnosed with breast cancer get somewhat clear treatment recommendations from their doctors: lumpectomy, chemotherapy, radiation, mastectomy, depending on the size and grade of the tumor. For a probably someday cancer, you get a long series of nearly impossible choices that no one can make easier for you.

The knowledge gives you the power to make decisions, but the choices aren't so great. For breast cancer, there's surveillance: regular mammograms alternating with MRI scans to try to catch any cancer early. Doctors say they *should* work. And they probably will. But there's no guarantee. Mammograms and MRIs can miss cancers, especially in younger women, who have denser breast tissue.

I could take a medication to lower the risk of cancer, called chemoprevention. It would come with a hefty price—early menopause.

Or, I could elect to have a major, major surgery that sounded unthinkable: a prophylactic bilateral mastectomy.

The choices aren't much better for protecting yourself from ovarian cancer. The recommendation is to have surgery to remove your fallopian tubes and both ovaries, called a risk-reducing bilateral salpingo-oophorectomy. There are no reliable tests to detect ovarian cancer at an early stage. Symptoms, which can include bloating or a feeling of fullness, can be easy to miss or easy to shrug off as something else. Most cases are not caught until the cancer has spread to other parts of the body. Only 20 percent of ovarian cancers are caught at an early stage, according to the American Cancer Society.[11] About 22,440 women were estimated to be diagnosed with ovarian cancer and 14,070 women were expected to die of ovarian cancer in 2018.[12]

So, the choices are not pretty. However, I'm grateful and I know I'm fortunate to have options. I wish my grandmother Lucy Belle and great-grandmother Margaret had had them. I feel lucky to live during the first time in history when high-risk women, at least those of us fortunate enough to have access to the testing, have at least a shot at overcoming our genetic destiny.

But I had no idea what to do. And no one could tell me.

CHAPTER 2

Not Simple, Pretty Things

"I choose not to keep my story private because there are many women who do not know that they might be living under the shadow of cancer. It is my hope that they, too, will be able to get gene tested, and that if they have a high risk they, too, will know that they have strong options.

Life comes with many challenges. The ones that should not scare us are the ones we can take on and take control of."

—Angelina Jolie, "My Medical Choice," *The New York Times* (2013)

How do you even begin to decide whether to have surgery to "remove" your breasts when you don't have cancer—and may never get it?

The idea of having a double mastectomy, especially having a double mastectomy to prevent breast cancer, completely freaked me out. Of course, so did the possibility of being diagnosed with and possibly dying of breast cancer. I had never had to deal with a potentially life-threatening medical issue or faced such an agonizing decision. I half wished my doctor would order me to have what I could only call The Surgery. (I couldn't utter the word "mastectomy.") I didn't want it to be something that I had to choose. A prophylactic double mastectomy, as the doctor called it, would be an elective surgery but I couldn't imagine electing to have one. About a year earlier, I had no trouble deciding to have my gallbladder taken out after an attack that had me doubled over on the bathroom floor in severe pain. My doctor recommended surgery. I went to the hospital, had the operation and was back at work a week later. The options for dealing with a BRCA mutation, however, were not so clear-cut. I could have surgery. Or not.

My doctors presented both as reasonable choices. Some women went with surgery; some used surveillance to manage their risk. There was no right or wrong answer, but I wanted the "right" one to appear in black and white. Instead it was somewhere inside a huge gray hole.

I was stuck with an annoying series of "what ifs" swirling in a twisted loop inside my head.

What if I go through the ordeal of surgery and losing my breasts but never was going to get cancer?

What if I go through the surgery and the next year, they discover a much simpler, less painful and invasive way to reduce my risk?

What if studies find that my cancer risk isn't so high after all?

What if I have the surgery and still get cancer?

What if I don't have the surgery and find out that cancer has spread throughout my body and that I've got six months to live?

What if? What if? What if? . . . I was driving myself crazy. Risk-reducing double mastectomy. Or close surveillance. When it comes down to it, the best option, well, it just depends.

I figured I would be a lot more likely to have a preventive surgery if a less conspicuous part of my body was at stake. I could deal with losing my appendix, my thyroid, or some other body part nobody, including myself, would notice. But we're talking about breasts here. Breasts, the bigger the better we are taught, are symbols of beauty, femininity, sexuality and motherhood. We grow up bombarded with messages that continue throughout our lives about how important boobs are in our culture: Barbies with supersized busts, *Baywatch*, any fashion or celebrity magazine, "breastaurant" chains and so-called "gentlemen's" clubs that cash in on the obsession. Writer Geralyn Lucas explored the phenomenon during a visit to a strip club to decide whether she could have a mastectomy in her book, *Why I Wore Lipstick to My Mastectomy*.

"All the men in this room are reminding me of the power I stand to lose. They are here to worship boobs. . . . a breast is somehow more than flesh and blood. Everywhere in life, but especially here. This is a crash course, a Cliffs Notes on why boobs matter so much. Men are paying a lot of money to look. And acting really stupid. Let's face it—they would not be behaving this way if the women were on stage pulling down their socks to reveal their ankles."[1]

If the girls didn't matter so much, breast augmentation would not be the No. 1 cosmetic surgical procedure, with more than 300,000 performed in the United States in 2017—more than 800 a day, according to the American Society of Plastic Surgeons.[2]

When comes down to it, breasts are just flesh and blood. Mine never seemed to carry the kind of special powers Lucas wrote about. But still, they were my breasts. Having them removed sounded traumatic. Faced with a life-threatening diagnosis, I wouldn't be able to get rid of them fast enough. If I'd been diagnosed with breast cancer—or if I knew my risk was closer to the high end of the estimates—I would schedule surgery as soon as possible. There wouldn't be any decision to make.

Dealing with a high risk of breast cancer, however, was not so clear cut. My doctor would not tell me that I should have a double mastectomy, only that I should consider one. Doctors, genetic counselors and the informational materials they gave me presented surveillance and surgery both as good approaches to managing my high risk.

So I was not in a rush to have The Surgery.

While a cancer diagnosis forces you to act, a BRCA mutation diagnosis gives you time to hesitate. I had no shortage of reasons, from practical to philosophical, to delay: *This isn't the right time. I can't take that much time off work right now. I need to save up enough money for the surgery. I need to do more research. I can't get my mind around having a double mastectomy. Maybe a better option will be developed soon. What if I go through all this pain and I was never going to get cancer anyway? Would I be scarred? Would I look or feel deformed? Would I always feel like I had strange uncomfortable foreign objects in my body? Would people think I was crazy?* If I had the surgery, there would be no going back.

Bottom line, I was not sold on surgery. My reluctance to embrace surgery may sound surprising to anyone who has read stories about women who quickly schedule surgery after discovering they have a BRCA mutation. However, few people had heard about BRCA mutations and preventative mastectomies in 2009, when I got my results. The idea of having this type of surgery was completely foreign to me. In fact, it sounded bizarre.

Many of the media stories about BRCA mutations focus on people with BRCA1 mutations, which carry a higher risk for breast cancer and a very aggressive type of breast cancer at that. If I had been diagnosed with a BRCA1 mutation, maybe I would have felt a greater sense of urgency. But my risk from a harmful BRCA2 mutation was lower than that of someone with a BRCA1 mutation, although it's impossible to say by how much. Some of the estimates put my risk at 45 percent, which, if true, would be nearly half that of a woman with a BRCA1 mutation. A roughly 50–50 chance of breast cancer was much different than almost certain odds. The problem was, I had no idea whether my risk was 45 percent or much higher.

What risk level reaches the threshold at which you should remove a healthy body part?

After learning they carry BRCA mutations, some women hurry and schedule preventative surgery because they have watched loved ones suffer and die from the horrible disease. Fortunately, that was not the case for me. My mom, in her late 60s, had never been diagnosed with breast cancer.

There was something else that held me back: I had what I now see as a naïve view about the threat of breast cancer. From what I understood at the time, if you get regular mammograms, you catch any breast cancer early, and if you catch cancer early, you get treated and go on to live a full life. The idea of breast cancer, while scary as hell, did not seem life-threatening as long as it was caught early. I had seen several women, including my mother-in-law, a supervisor, and my friend's mom, survive breast cancer and thrive. I thought the danger only came if you did not catch breast cancer before it had spread to other parts of the body. I was told that my grandmother and great-grand-mother were too scared to go to a doctor until it was too late. Early detection was the key, I thought. I did not know anything about the different types of breast cancers and that some were more aggressive than others. I had no idea that, while early detection saves lives, it does not come with a guarantee.

The more I read about BRCA mutations and breast cancer, the more I realized I needed to learn. If I was supposed to consider having a double mastectomy, I was going to do my homework.

Tangled in my fear and confusion were messages that The Surgery was drastic, extreme, unnecessary and even misguided.

I found out about my BRCA2 mutation four years before actress Angelina Jolie announced her own risk-reducing double mastectomy in 2013. Most people, including me, knew little, if anything, at the time about BRCA mutations or double mastectomies to reduce breast cancer risk. I worried that people would think I was crazy to have my breasts removed. How would my then-husband feel about me having fake boobs, or no boobs? He was as confused about the whole thing as I was and encouraged me to research and understand my options.

When I told a handful of people that my doctor recommended I consider this option, I got "the look": the look where their eyes go wide and their necks jet back as if you just told them something horrible and shocking like, well, that you are considering having your breasts removed. I got a few comments about how that seemed drastic and was I sure it was necessary?

"Surgeons just want to cut," my mom said when I first told her my breast surgeon suggested I consider a double mastectomy.

It felt like nobody understood the risks I faced. In addition to the psychological and physical pain of surgery and losing my breasts, I worried about judgment, or at the very least, a lack of support. The few initial reactions I got made me want to keep the whole thing to myself. Mostly, that's what I did.

At least I knew I wasn't alone. In a magazine interview, Jessica Queller, author of the memoir *Pretty Is What Changes* and TV writer who worked on the wonderful *Gilmore Girls,* shared the negative reactions she received about having a prophylactic mastectomy at age 35 due to a BRCA1 mutation.

"People were very judgmental. Everyone from my friends to strangers online. So many people posted things online after this 'Nightline' interview that I did, saying things like, 'Please, Jessica, don't do it. You could get hit by a bus tomorrow, you never know.' One guy wrote, 'I can't believe she's doing this. It's the equivalent of being castrated.'"[3]

Miss D.C. Allyn Rose also faced judgment when she announced in 2012 that she was having a double mastectomy to reduce her risk of breast cancer, which had killed her mother at a young age.[4] In a TED talk at Chapman University, Rose said she received hate mail over her decision.

"People were pretty offended," she said.[5] "You have people who say, 'Don't have the surgery. This is mutilating your body. You don't have cancer.' They want to pick apart every little thing."

Angelina Jolie became a hero to women at high risk of hereditary breast and ovarian cancer when she wrote in *The New York Times* in May 2013[6] about her decision to have a double mastectomy to reduce her risk of cancer because she carries a BRCA1 mutation. In her *New York Times* article, thoughtfully titled "My Medical Choice," Jolie said she decided to have the surgery to be proactive to minimize her risk as much as possible. She emphasized that her choice isn't the only option for women at high risk of breast cancer. She wrote that each woman facing hereditary breast cancer risk should determine what is right for her.

"I wanted to write this to tell other women that the decision to have a mastectomy was not easy. But it is one I am very happy that I made. My chances of developing breast cancer have dropped from 87 percent to under 5 percent. I can tell my children that they don't need to fear they will lose me to breast cancer."

The article took some of the stigma and mystery out of prophylactic mastectomies and raised awareness about genetic testing. Here was one of the most beautiful women in the world showing that women can still look and feel attractive after a double mastectomy. "On a personal note, I do not feel any less of a woman. I feel empowered that I made a strong choice that in no way diminishes my femininity," Jolie wrote.

Suddenly everyone was talking about this thing that no one seemed to understand just a day earlier. I hoped that by opening up about her experience, Jolie would help people see The Surgery as not so bizarre. Then, maybe I wouldn't be quite so scared or weirded out about it. Jolie received an outpouring of support. There was judgment, too. Some so-called "experts" and readers claimed that Jolie's surgery was not necessary, as if women who undergo preventative mastectomies are duped by scalpel-happy surgeons. There were concerns that the news would encourage other women to "maim" or "mutilate" themselves, as if women would rush out to have double mastectomies to be like Jolie. Others characterized Jolie's surgery as a Hollyweird thing or an "elite" surgery only available to a wealthy celebrity rather than something insurance plans cover because it costs them less to prevent than to treat cancer.

The news headlines that followed Jolie's disclosure demonstrated the lack of understanding about the level of risk that comes with BRCA mutations:

"Angelina Jolie's double mastectomy fueling national debate"[7]—ABC News

"More women opting for preventative mastectomy—but should they be?"[8]—NBC News

NBC also ran the story: "Doctors Approve of Angelina Jolie's Surgery" after Jolie had her ovaries removed in 2015.[9]

Although many called Jolie courageous, singer Melissa Etheridge, who publicly battled breast cancer and said she also has a BRCA mutation, took issue with that characterization in a widely publicized interview with the *Washington Blade*.[10] The

Blade asked Etheridge, as a cancer survivor, what she thought of Jolie's announcement. Her response was:

> I have to say I feel a little differently. I have that gene mutation too and it's not something I would believe in for myself. I wouldn't call it the brave choice. I actually think it's the most fearful choice you can make when confronting anything with cancer. My belief is that cancer comes from inside you and so much of it has to do with the environment of your body. It's the stress that will turn that gene on or not. Plenty of people have the gene mutation and everything but it never comes to cancer so I would say to anybody faced with that, that choice is way down the line on the spectrum of what you can do and to really consider the advancements we've made in things like nutrition and stress levels. I've been cancer free for nine years now and looking back, I completely understand why I got cancer. There was so much acidity in everything. I really encourage people to go a lot longer and further before coming to that conclusion.[11]

Besides her controversial claims about the role of stress or acidity in cancer, Etheridge's comments reflected the kind of thinking that fueled my own anxiety about making the wrong decision—and about how people would react if I had the surgery.

Along with misinformation came violent and frightening language to describe mastectomies. Some websites and commenters on news sites described the surgery as mutilation and used language about women "lopping," "cutting" or "chopping" off their breasts as if a surgeon took a knife and sliced off each breast from top to bottom. Perhaps this language goes back to the days of radical mastectomies, known as the Halsted mastectomy, that left women disfigured by taking out large chunks of tissue including muscle and lymph nodes. Thankfully, mastectomies have changed, and radical mastectomies are no longer the standard of care. Surgeons no longer take out muscle and they leave as many lymph nodes as possible, depending on whether and how far cancer, if there is any, has spread. Instead, depending on the type of mastectomy, surgeons can make an incision that is much smaller than I imagined, a few inches in some cases, remove the breast tissue and replace it with implants or expanders if the patient wants reconstruction. Plastic surgeons also can create beautiful new breasts using more natural feeling tissue from patients' stomach, back or butt. High-risk women who have not had breast cancer often can keep their nipples. If that's not possible, they can become the girl with the nipple tattoo. There are talented tattoo specialists who can create new ones with an amazing 3D effect.

The words used to describe mastectomy matter. Creating an incision and removing abnormal breast tissue sounds less threatening than "chopping off your breasts"—and it's the truth. The Surgery began to seem a little less scary when I began to think of it in those terms. Harsh, violent rhetoric fuels stigma, controversy and fear over the surgery and could keep women from taking steps that could save their lives. No one wants to have to deal with something like this or have to think about it. But the hostile reactions toward women who choose prophylactic bilateral mastectomies reveal more than a deep discomfort with cancer or the idea of the surgery. I mean, you don't hear anyone telling a woman she mutilated herself by having a problem thyroid removed.

In her book, *A Cancer in the Family: Take Control of Your Genetic Inheritance*, Dr. Theodora Ross wrote about how the negative reactions to Jolie's surgery were based in fear. "When the actress Angelina Jolie publicly announced that she had a

BRCA1 mutation and had decided to undergo prophylactic mastectomies, people felt anxious—even those people without a family history of cancer. To justify this anxiety, they engaged in their own form of denial, which unfortunately can look a lot like criticism or blaming. That's why, in the days after Jolie's announcement, you heard people 'explaining' why she didn't really need the surgery or suggesting that she was going to lead a trend in unnecessary procedures. These were people who weren't ready to accept that Jolie had made intelligent, powerful decisions that probably saved her life," wrote Ross, professor of internal medicine and director of the Genetics Program in the Harold C. Simmons Comprehensive Cancer Center at the University of Texas Southwestern Medical Center.[12]

The criticism about Jolie making a "fearful" decision struck a nerve because I didn't want to make my decision out of fear (and I don't believe that Jolie did). I wanted to make the best decision for my peace of mind and for my family. On the other hand, how could fear not be a factor? I had a lot of it. I was afraid of getting cancer. Of dying young just like my grandmother and great-grandmother. I was afraid of what suddenly seemed like a real possibility of not seeing my son grow up . . . I could go on. There was no way to untangle fear from the decision. I was scared to have a prophylactic double mastectomy. I was scared of not having one.

To make a smart decision, I needed more information. I approached my BRCA research as I would as a reporter digging into a big story. It helped distract me. One of the first things I wondered was, what do other women in this situation do? As with a lot of my questions, the research was limited because

BRCA was so new. The few studies I found indicated that most women with BRCA mutations do not have preventative mastectomies, at least within five years of being tested.

A 2012 study in the journal *International Journal of Cancer* found that 36 percent of a sample of U.S. women who tested positive for BRCA 1 or BRCA2 mutations had prophylactic bilateral mastectomies within 5.3 years after testing.[13] (The study also found that 71 percent of those women had risk-reducing bilateral salpingo-oophorectomies.) Public awareness about BRCA and risk-reducing surgery has increased since the study was conducted, which was done before Angelina Jolie's article, so it's possible that the numbers have changed.

Rates of preventative mastectomies among women with BRCA mutations varied from country to country, with the U.S. having the highest, according to another study.[14] Holland was close behind, with about one in three high-risk women opting for prophylactic mastectomies. In France, it was one in four women; in Italy, one in 10; and fewer than 1 in 20 in Norway.[15] The study is one of few available, however, on this topic. It's unclear how and whether factors such as cost, insurance, availability of surgery or physicians' attitudes played a role in the number of surgeries.

Regardless of people's attitudes about the surgery, there's plenty of evidence that it works. Multiple studies have found that the procedure cuts a BRCA mutation carrier's risk of breast cancer below that of the average woman.[16] The Society of Surgical Oncology Breast Disease Working Group published a review of existing research that highlighted these findings. The group of surgical oncologists concluded that women with BRCA mutations who have bilateral prophylactic mastectomies and who have their ovaries removed reduce their risk of breast cancer by 95 percent.[17]

"From the published data, it is clear that BPM (bilateral prophylactic mastectomy) confers a reduction in the risk of developing a primary breast cancer approaching 100 percent when meticulous surgical technique is used to remove a vast majority of breast tissue," the authors wrote.[18]

The lead author, Kelly Hunt, M.D., chair and professor, department of breast surgical oncology, division of surgery, at The University of Texas MD Anderson Cancer Center in Houston, said in an interview for this book that she advises patients with BRCA mutations who are trying to make decisions to start by talking to their genetic counselor and physicians to understand their cancer risk as much as possible. Hunt emphasized that risk is not static. It can change, for example, if a patient has a relative who is diagnosed with cancer or if the patient has a biopsy that reveals an abnormal cell growth such as atypical ductal hyperplasia.[19]

"I try to understand my patients' family history because the age of diagnosis of breast cancer of different family members can certainly influence the timing of any risk-reducing surgery they're planning to do," Hunt said. For example, a patient with a BRCA mutation whose mother was diagnosed with breast cancer in her 30s may consider having a prophylactic bilateral mastectomy by the time she turns 30. Younger women have the added difficulty of factoring in their desire to have or finish having children to the timing of any surgeries. Hunt also suggests that patients visit a plastic surgeon early on.

"It's good to get an understanding of what the reconstructive options are and then help patients navigate the really challenging process of changes in body image because the reconstructive surgery, while excellent, is not going to make the patient look exactly like they did before, and that can be challenging for women to navigate as well. How are they going to look and feel afterwards, what's life going to look like after the surgery—those are all really important things that we work through in planning any type of surgical intervention," Hunt said. She said there are tradeoffs to consider in any course of action: Surgery comes with risks and potential complications and surveillance has its pros and cons, so each patient must decide what works best for them.

As genetic links continue to be discovered that can warn us about various cancers and other diseases, more and more of us will face difficult decisions about our health. How far can and should we go to prevent disease after we discover we have a hereditary risk? Which body parts or organs are we willing to live without? What are the consequences of sacrificing our breasts or ovaries? How much control do we actually have over the instructions coded into our genes? Medical advances undoubtedly will give us better choices down the road. We may be able to fix the genetic mutation one day. For now, though, the science is way ahead of the solutions, like a fairy godmother who appears before the wand has been invented.

Scientists continue to discover more genes linked to hereditary cancers, including breast cancer, that expand the decisions beyond those of us with BRCA1 or BRCA2 mutations. There's *ATM, CDH1, CHEK2, MRE11A, NBN, PALB2, PTEN, RAD50, RAD51C,* and *TP53, to name a few.*[20] Each of these mutations carries a different level of risk (and some of these risks are still being determined) and some of these genetic mutations also carry risks for other diseases. Every year at a Dallas one-day conference on hereditary cancer, genetic counselors discuss new inherited genetic links as the science continues to unfold. These genetic mutations connect the dots for families who've watched generations of loved ones die of cancer.

After Angelina Jolie wrote about her high risk and double mastectomy, countless worried women asked their doctors if they, too, should be tested for what many were calling the "breast cancer gene." There is no such thing as a "breast cancer gene." Everyone has two sets of BRCA1 and BRCA2 genes that are supposed to protect us from breast cancer. The high risk comes when a person has a mutation, or variance in one of the genes. A 2016 study in the journal *BMJ* documented a 64 percent increase in testing among women ages 18 to 64 in the two weeks after the editorial.[21] There was no such spike during the same period in the previous year, according to the study. Despite the increased concern about hereditary breast and ovarian cancer, most women have nothing to worry about. Most breast cancers are not hereditary.

BRCA mutations affect a small percentage of the population. But most of the people who have them do not know it. A 2012 study in the *Annals of Surgical Oncology* estimated that 941,155 U.S. women and men carry a BRCA mutation, with 348,274 of them being women over age 20.[22] At the time of the study, the researchers estimated that only a fraction of estimated mutation carriers—48,754—had been identified. While BRCA testing allows women to make decisions that can help them prevent breast and ovarian cancer, too many women do not discover that they have a BRCA mutation until *after* a cancer diagnosis. Although it's too late to prevent their cancer, the knowledge can help them make decisions to try to prevent another cancer. The positive result also can serve as a signal that other family members should talk to a genetic counselor about whether they, too, should be tested.

The nonprofit organization dedicated to hereditary breast and ovarian cancer, Facing Our Risk of Cancer Empowered (FORCE) recommends that women with a strong family history of cancer should consult with a genetic counselor, especially if they or a relative have had any of the following:[23]

- ovarian, fallopian tube, or primary peritoneal cancer
- breast cancer at age 50 or younger
- two separate breast cancers
- a type of breast cancer called "triple negative breast cancer"
- male breast cancer
- pancreatic cancer
- prostate cancer at age 55 or younger or metastatic prostate cancer (cancer that spread outside the prostate)
- Eastern European Jewish ancestry and any of the above cancers at any age

Or, if more than one family member on the same side of your family has had:

- breast cancer
- ovarian, fallopian tube, primary peritoneal cancer
- prostate cancer
- pancreatic cancer

Some experts have raised concerns that limiting testing to those who meet certain family history criteria may leave out too many people who could have a high risk for hereditary breast and ovarian cancer. Dr. Mary-Claire King, the pioneering geneticist who identified the section of chromosome 17 that carried particular genetic markers for women with breast cancer in severely affected families, has advocated that all women be tested.

"I believe that every woman should be offered testing of BRCA1 and BRCA2 at about age 30 as part of routine medical care. About half of women who inherit mutations in BRCA1 or BRCA2 have no family history of breast or ovarian cancer and have no idea they are carrying cancer-causing mutations," Dr. King told *The New York Times*. "Most inherited breast and ovarian cancer can be prevented, if mutation carriers know who they are. Granted, the solution is not pretty. It requires removing the ovaries and fallopian tubes by about age 40 to eliminate almost all the ovarian cancer risk and to reduce breast cancer risk by about half. Some women opt also for prophylactic mastectomy to reduce the breast cancer risk almost to zero."[24]

King and several co-authors conducted a study that tested 8,000 healthy men in the Ashkenazi Jewish population of Israel. Half of those who tested positive for a BRCA mutation had no close family history that would have triggered attention.[25] Many have no idea whether there was a family history of cancer and no relatives to ask since entire families were killed in the horror of the Holocaust.

There are other reasons some people may not be aware of their risk. Some families are small, resulting in less obvious cancer patterns. Families that are not in touch may not know about cancers that have affected distant relatives. Some women inherit BRCA mutations from their fathers, who may have no sisters or no history of family breast cancer that would raise red flags. BRCA testing has unearthed another issue—some families have secret histories that can leave people unaware of their potential risk. Some people may be unaware of their Ashkenazi Jewish heritage, which would put them at higher risk. The long, ugly history of anti-Semitism forced people to change their identities in the past. In her book, Ross wrote about how she discovered an unknown ethnic history in her own family after she tested positive for a BRCA1 mutation common in Ashkenazi Jewish populations. Initially, she thought the mutation came from her father because his side of her family was Jewish and had a history of cancer. She was surprised when she learned that it came from her mother's side of the family. Her mother was Catholic, and her family had immigrated to the United States from Poland near the end of World War I.[26] Unknown ethnic histories can give some people a false sense of security about their risk or have them looking for answers on the wrong branch of the family tree.

My own family history wouldn't have necessarily set off alerts for genetic testing. The first risk assessment tool (before I tested positive for a BRCA mutation), which put me at an 18 percent risk, did not flag me as higher risk because I did not have a first-degree relative diagnosed with breast cancer. As a result, I had a false sense of security.

Some people don't want to know if they carry a BRCA mutation, which is understandable. In a 2016 article in *Wired*, science writer Cynthia Graeber wrote that a positive test would not convince her to get surgery. "It would just feel like hefting a sword, dangling it by a frayed thread above my head, and waiting for it to fall. I'm more scared of living like that than I am of cancer," she wrote.[27]

I wouldn't want to know that I have a genetic predisposition for a disease that I couldn't do anything about. With BRCA mutations, though, patients can make choices that could save their lives. The important thing is that we can become informed and make the best decisions for ourselves, as difficult as they may be. Like Dr. Mary-Claire King said, the choices are "not simple, pretty things."

How would I decide whether to remove a rather important body part without knowing whether it may or may not save my life? I realized that the biggest hurdle was psychological.

I mean, I never worried about whether I'd still be desirable without my gallbladder.

CHAPTER 3

The Fault in Our Genes

"Ask questions, that's all I've ever tried to do since day one. My advice is be involved in your care, dot your i's and cross your t's. Take control. And talk with other patients. They can help you."[1]

—Annie Parker, BRCA1 mutation carrier, three-time cancer survivor, author of *Annie Parker Decoded*

had opened Pandora's box. Now, I needed to look deeper inside.

The first thing I wanted to know was: Could the test could be wrong? The answer was, probably not. Only one company, Myriad Genetics in Utah, offered BRCA mutation analysis when I was tested in 2009. Myriad had a patent on the test because the company discovered the precise sequence of the BRCA1 and BRCA2 genes linked to hereditary breast and ovarian cancer. (The U.S. Supreme Court ruled in 2013 that Myriad could not patent a naturally occurring gene segment, which allowed other companies to provide the test.)[2]

I searched online for stories of women with false positives. I didn't find any. Some people received ambiguous results, and many women with family histories of breast cancer were surprised to get negative results. The test is known for having a high accuracy rate. Still, I didn't know how seriously to take this BRCA stuff at the time. I read obsessively about the issue. I devoured everything I could find about BRCA mutations on the Internet, medical journal articles and the few books that were available at the time. Looking back, I think I was searching for information that would provide a way out, a way to not have to take this so seriously. I hoped to hear that the BRCA mutation risk was overblown. Maybe BRCA wasn't as big of a deal as my doctors made it seem. Instead of finding evidence to help me stuff BRCA back in that box, the message kept coming at me: This BRCA stuff is real. I had been somewhat in denial. Denial is the first stage of grief, as the theory by Elisabeth Kübler-Ross and David Kessler goes. It seemed to be my favorite, since I hung onto it for so long! I had no reason to doubt my test result, especially given my family history. The next step would be for my mom and two sisters to get tested for the mutation. We made an appointment with a genetic counselor my mom and I had met and liked at a local conference on hereditary breast and ovarian cancer.

BRCA mutations can be inherited from either parent. If my mom had the genetic mutation, and I was betting that she did, my sisters and I each had a 50/50 chance of inheriting it from her. Given the history of breast cancers on my mom's side, it would have been a shock if she did not test positive for the same BRCA2 mutation. Since my test had pinpointed the exact location of the mutation on the gene, my mom and sisters could get simpler and much less expensive tests (about $300 each at that time) that checked for the same mutation: 8803delC.

None of us had problems getting insurance to cover the test, thankfully, given our family history. BRCA testing had become a standard thing to warrant insurance coverage when a patient demonstrated various risk factors. I worry about people who do not have any insurance or inadequate coverage. The Affordable Care Act mandated coverage of genetic testing for patients that meet certain criteria.[3] And there are some nonprofits that help.

My mom and sisters and I met with a genetic counselor on a weekday afternoon. Once again, I left work for another medical appointment. I was missing a lot of work to go to all these doctors' visits. Before the BRCA test, I rarely used any sick time. I was lucky I had built up a lot of it, but I still felt guilty for taking time off work. The five of us sat at a round office table in a small, stuffy windowless conference room with blank white walls. I gave her a copy of my Myriad lab report and she took down information about our family history. She explained some basics about genetics and the BRCA gene. She said my grandmother, great-grandmother, great aunts and great uncle probably had the mutation, given their cancer histories. My mom asked a lot of questions.

"If my mother and grandmother had this, why wouldn't I have gotten cancer yet?" she asked.

"You may have inherited other genes that helped protect you against cancer," she said. After we talked for about an hour, my mom and sisters went down the hall to have blood drawn and sent to Myriad.

The results came in about a week later. My mom and sisters and I met with the counselor again. The news was no surprise to any of us. My mom had the mutation. Unfortunately, so did one of my sisters. The good news was that my other sister did not. The counselor created a diagram of our family history. Seeing it on paper made it look even worse. Our genetic counselor, like the one I originally went to, put the news in a positive light. It would allow us to do something about our broken-down gene. The test would give us the documentation we needed for insurance providers to approve enhanced screenings. We could be proactive. We hugged each other goodbye after the appointment. Then I had to get back to work. I had to file it away, to obsess and worry about later, so I could get through the rest of my work day.

So, there it was. The tests confirmed what we already knew was probably true. Now what?

My mom and sisters' tests made the BRCA mutation seem a little more real. It was starting to feel even more serious. I had so many questions I needed to answer to help me figure out what to do. Did women who chose double mastectomies have any regrets? How well does surveillance work—what are the chances that close screenings could still miss a tumor? Which option would give me the best chance of living a long, healthy life?

The more research I did, the more questions I had. When you're trying to make a major life decision, you want to know the stakes. As with all things BRCA, that's not always easy to pin down. It felt like I was trying to make this huge, life-altering decision partially blindfolded. There was no way to truly know my risk of getting breast and/or ovarian cancer beyond a wide range of numbers that are simply estimates. If my risk was 45 percent or 50 percent, and I had surgery to remove my ovaries, which lowers breast cancer risk by 50 percent, would that lower my total risk to 25 percent? And if I eat a perfect diet and exercise regularly, would that lower my risk even more?

The estimates are a range because they come from various studies that involved different populations. Also, not all BRCA mutations are alike. Mutations occur at different locations on the BRCA1 or BRCA2 genes, and each may carry different risks. One of the most comprehensive studies in a top medical journal, a 2017 *Journal of the American Medical Association* (*JAMA*) study of 10,000 women with BRCA1 and BRCA2 mutations, estimated the following risk by age 80:[4]

BRCA1 mutation carriers:

- 72 percent risk of breast cancer
- 44 percent risk of ovarian cancer

BRCA2 mutation carriers:

- 69 percent risk of breast cancer
- 17 percent risk of ovarian cancer

The study found that the risk of breast cancer in the other breast within 20 years of a breast cancer diagnosis was 40 percent for women with BRCA1 mutations and 26 percent for women with BRCA2 mutations.[5]

Family history is also critical for evaluating your risk for breast and ovarian cancer. The *JAMA* study found that the risk of breast cancer in BRCA1 and BRCA2 carriers increased based on the number of relatives who had been diagnosed with breast cancer.[6] Based on my own grim family history, I worried that my risk was at the high end of those estimates. Few, if any, relatives who appear to have inherited the BRCA mutation escaped cancer.

After doing some research, we found that at least seven people within three generations of our family died of cancers associated with BRCA2 mutations.

The first that I know of was my great-great grandmother, Ida Belle. She died at age 85 of what we had been told was a stomach cancer. After we discovered that the BRCA2 mutation carries increased risks for not only breast cancer but also ovarian and pancreatic cancer, we wondered if Ida Belle's "stomach" cancer could have been ovarian cancer, which nobody would have talked about when she died in the late 1960s. Our family is pretty sure the mutation was passed down from her, because cancer did not run in my great-great grandfather's family. My mom looked up Ida Belle's death certificate. She found the true cause of death: pancreatic cancer, making it likely that she carried the BRCA2 mutation.

The BRCA2 mutation took a huge toll on Ida Belle's six children. Five of them—three daughters and two sons—died of cancer when they were in their 40s and 50s.

Cancer struck them one by one.

My great-grandmother, Margaret, was the first to become ill. Margaret, who I picture in black and white and from the side because of the angle in one of the few photos I've seen of her, was diagnosed with breast cancer in her early 40s. She had felt a lump for months, but was too scared to go to the doctor, according to my mom, whose mother told her about it. By the time she finally got medical help, the cancer was eating through the skin on her breast. Her doctor found that the tumor had spread throughout her body. Margaret had radiation, but it was too late.

Margaret died of breast cancer in 1943 when she was only 46. She had two children. One of them was my grandmother, who was in her early 20s when she had to watch her mom go through an excruciating death.

Margaret's sister, Betty, was the second daughter in that family to be diagnosed with cancer. She died in 1959, two years after her diagnosis. She was in her mid-50s. My mom, who was 14 at the time, was devastated. Betty was her favorite great-aunt, the one who had doted on her and taken her shopping. No one told my mom at the time that Betty had died of cancer. People didn't talk about cancer back then. As my mom says, this was a time when people said someone was "PG" instead of pregnant and married couples on TV slept in separate twin beds. When my mom was older, she was told that Betty had died of liver cancer. While Betty's cancer may have metastasized to her liver, we only recently found evidence that it did not begin there. We now know the truth that no one was willing to tell my mom when she was a young teen-ager. My mom recently looked up Betty's death certificate, which states that she died of "pelvic carcinoma" and "pelvic lymphoma." My mom confirmed with a relative: Betty had died of ovarian cancer. We never knew that we had any cases of ovarian cancer in our family until after we learned about our BRCA2 mutation. The silence and stigma surrounding cancer in the 1950s and 1960s kept us from understanding the reality of our risk sooner. The fact that it was more acceptable to say that Betty died of liver cancer than ovarian cancer kept our family and many others in the dark about their risk and allowed an awful family history to repeat itself.

Next, Myrtle, Margaret and Betty's sister, got sick. She, too, was diagnosed with a pelvic cancer that we now suspect was ovarian cancer. She only lived a few years, also dying in her early 40s, leaving behind a son.

The fourth sister, Katherine, was the most fortunate. She lived into her 70s. She didn't dodge cancer, though. She was the only one of my great-great aunts who was still alive when I was a kid. I remember playing at her house, going to lunch with her at a cafeteria and thinking she was very old. I remember her talking about how bloated her illness had made her become. I remembered being told she had stomach cancer. After we discovered the BRCA2 mutation in our family, we speculated that she may have had ovarian cancer. Then, after finding her death certificate, we discovered that she died of a different BRCA2-related cancer: "pancreatic carcinoma." (We also discovered that her son died of pancreatic cancer in 2014 when he was in his 70s.)

One of the brothers in that generation died of cancer as well. We don't know what type. He was only in his 50s, which suggests it could have been another BRCA2-related cancer because it struck at a younger-than-average age. The other son died of a heart attack at 85. Five out of six children in that family died of cancer. I would bet that each of them inherited the BRCA2 mutation. Why did three daughters die in their 40s while one did not get cancer until into her 70s? Why did one son not get cancer? Did he not have the mutation? Or did he have a genetic mutation that never resulted in cancer? We'll never know.

The BRCA2 mutation took a tremendous toll on the next generation.

Margaret had five children: three girls and two boys. At least two of them appear to have inherited the BRCA2 mutation.

One of them was my grandmother, Lucy Belle. She was born in 1921 and grew up and raised her family in Kansas City. During World War II, my grandmother worked in a war munitions factory making bullets, just like Rosie the Riveter. My mom describes her as loving, fun and sometimes silly. She also suffered from anxiety (which also runs in my family) and was in a very unhappy marriage. My mom, Linda, was only 15 when she found Lucy Belle, who was only 38 at the time, crying. Her mom told her that she had a lump in her breast and would need a mastectomy. They were the only ones in their small house that day. My mom had never heard of cancer until that moment. That's when her mom told her that her dear aunt Betty had died of cancer and that Lucy Belle's mother, Margaret, had died young of breast cancer. Margaret died the year before my mom was born.

"The first thing I remember asking her was 'How long have you had it?'" my mom said. Lucy Belle had felt something for six months but did not tell anyone or see a doctor. "She told me she was scared and had not confided in anyone until she knew it was not going away." After seeing her own mother die of breast cancer, Lucy Belle must have been terrified. In those days, cancer was surrounded by stigma and felt more like a death sentence.

Once she went to the doctor, Lucy Belle's treatment marked the standard of care at that time. In 1961, shortly after her diagnosis, she had a radical mastectomy and radiation. A radical mastectomy is just what the term implies. Surgeons routinely removed patients' entire breast, surrounding tissue, lymph nodes and pectoral muscles. The operation left Lucy Belle with scars to her elbows where lymph nodes had been removed. The radiation left her skin red with horrible, painful burns that looked like she had been scalded. My mom, who was in high school, took care of the household because her mother's surgery left her weak and in constant pain. Two years after the mastectomy, Lucy Belle began having severe pain. The doctors found the cancer had spread to her bones. She had more radiation and more excruciating pain during her last months. She was in the hospital when mom graduated from high school. My mom worked in the bookkeeping department of a bank after she graduated. The hospital eventually sent Lucy Belle home, saying there was nothing else they could do for her. My mom quit her job to take care of Lucy Belle. She sat with her as much as possible, holding her hand and talking to her. By this time, cancer had moved to Lucy Belle's brain. My mom said she was the only person her mother recognized in her last few days of life. My mom was at her side when she took her last breath.

Lucy Belle died on Nov. 1, 1963, leaving my devastated mom and her two devastated brothers, ages 9 and 15.

My mom said she was hurt and confused about why no friends or relatives came to help when her mother was sick. Here was a young girl taking care of her two younger brothers and dying mother while their father would be gone for weeks at a time. However, at that time, people didn't know how cancer spread so they kept away from anyone who had it. People did not think cancer was hereditary. Fear and stigma about cancer not only contributed to my grandmother's horrible early death but made the situation even more painful and difficult for her family by leaving them to face the tragedy alone.

After her mother's death, my mom was beginning to understand the extent of the damage that cancer had caused in her family. Lucy Belle's brother, Eddie, also died of breast cancer. He was 68. My great uncle served in the U.S. Air Force in Korea. A male with breast cancer should be a bright red flashing flag that could signal a genetic mutation in a family. (While hereditary breast cancer often strikes women at younger ages than other breast cancers, it often does not affect men until later in their lives.)

Lucy Belle and Eddie may have been the only siblings in that generation of the family to have the BRCA2 mutation. One of their sisters died from kidney disease when she was only eight. Their brother committed suicide in his 70s. (Depression also runs in our family.) The third sister remains alive and healthy into her 90s. While it's possible to have a BRCA mutation and not get cancer, I doubt that was the case for the few relatives in my maternal family tree who died of other causes. My great-great uncle who did not die of cancer had two sons who never had cancer, which would be unlikely if all of them carried the mutation. The lack of any incidences of cancer in those relatives is a strong indication that they did not inherit the BRCA mutation.

Lucy Belle had two sons and a daughter. One son, my uncle, tested positive for the BRCA2 mutation a few years ago. He survived bladder cancer and died at age 67 from health problems that were unrelated to the BRCA2 mutation. My other uncle has not been tested.

Learning more about our family tree made me more worried than ever about my odds. I also had to consider my own history. Like a lot of women, I had fibrocystic breasts, which means that cysts, or fluid-filled sacs, come and go, especially around my period. It makes the self-exams they tell you to do pretty difficult. I was scared that if I had a tumor, I would never know. I'd already had that one breast cancer scare, with the biopsy that found atypical ductal hyperplasia.

"You should've been watched closely after that," Dr. A told me. However, my doctor at the time told me I simply needed to get regular mammograms.

The problem with finding out about the mutation was that I felt like I needed to do something about it. Before I made any decisions, I wanted second, third and maybe even fourth opinions. I had consultations with several doctors because I needed more input. Looking back, I think I was trying to find a reason, any reason, to not choose what I could only call The Surgery. I still couldn't say the M-word: mastectomy. Instead, I would tell doctors I wanted to understand my risk and my options, without using that frightening word.

Over the next several months, I met with several breast surgeons and gynecological oncologists. Every step of dealing with a BRCA mutation raised new questions that required more research. I talked to people involved in the local FORCE support group and connected with women on the FORCE message boards to get recommendations for doctors in Dallas who had experience with preventative surgeries. I searched for information about each doctor online, including looking up their profiles on the Texas Medical Board website to see what schools they went to and when and to make sure they had never been the subject of any disciplinary actions.

That led me to Dr. C, a gynecological oncologist. He came recommended from two different sources. We talked in his office, him behind a dark wood desk with stacks of journals and papers. Like Dr. A, he said mastectomy was a personal decision. He strongly encouraged me to have a bilateral salpingo-oophorectomy, a procedure that removed ovaries and fallopian tubes. He even suggested that I have the double mastectomies and bilateral salpingo-oophorectomy in one surgery. This was the first time I had heard of the option to do both surgeries at once. I didn't know that was possible. It sounded horrible.

"Uh. I'm not quite ready for that," I said. I asked if there was an advantage to having both surgeries at once. He said that fewer surgeries means less risk. Plus, you're done.

It was too much for me to consider at the time.

I asked him what he would recommend to a family member in my situation.

"Statistically, you're probably going to get breast cancer," he said. "Prevention is always better than treating an illness. With preventative surgery, you take control of the situation."

I said I was sure I'd have a bilateral salpingo-oophorectomy but that I could not get my mind around the mastectomies.

"The bilateral salpingo-oophorectomy is actually a tougher surgery from a recovery standpoint," he said. "Your body has to adjust to the loss of hormones. But the breast surgery is harder for most women."

Dr. C was sympathetic. He said he understood the difficulty of deciding to have a double mastectomy. He recommended a breast surgeon for me to talk to, one who has worked with him on the two-in-one procedure. I scheduled an appointment. Each appointment meant another $40 copay. I had no idea if my insurance would pay for all these consultations. The charges were adding up. All the doctors' offices started to look alike. Another bland waiting room. Another stiff light blue paper vest/gown.

The breast surgeon he recommended was young, good-looking and had long hair for a doctor. He was more emphatic about the breast surgery than the other doctors I'd seen so far.

"You need to do this surgery."

I was sitting on an exam table, rocking my paper vest.

"You're definitely a good candidate for nipple-sparing, skin-sparing mastectomies."

There was that nipple-sparing talk again.

I'd been wanting someone to tell me what to do, to make these decisions easier. Now, finally, here was a surgeon telling me I should have a double mastectomy. My muscles tensed up as if someone had made me drink an anxiety shot. My mind was saying wait a minute, not so fast, Doctor.

"I just can't get my head around having surgery to remove healthy tissue," I said out of frustration with the whole ordeal. The idea of surgery was driving me crazy. Having a double mastectomy to prevent a cancer I may never get felt so counterintuitive. I was not sick. How could I ever make peace with having The Surgery when I might never get cancer in the first place?

Dr. D paused before he spoke.

"But your tissue is not healthy. It has an abnormality that makes it unable to protect you from breast cancer."

I hadn't heard anyone put it that way. He had a point. My tissue wasn't healthy.

Dr. D's comment made me shift my thinking about my "healthy" breasts. Here was a doctor telling me that yes, I should have this surgery. Isn't that what I wanted? I still knew I didn't have to. And I was desperate to find another way out.

A friend recommended I talk to a doctor into alternative medicine. I loved the idea of taking a more "natural" approach and finding a way to address my cancer risk without surgery. Our first "meeting" was a phone consultation that cost me around $200. The doctor didn't accept insurance, but I could submit a claim to my insurance company.

My schedule was crammed that day. I ended up speaking to the doctor in a parking lot before an assignment. I remember sitting in my old gray Camry parked in a townhome complex. I was about to interview Mack, a homeless man who had lived in a cardboard box under a downtown freeway bridge for 17 years. That day, he was moving into a townhome purchased by a nonprofit organization. I first met him when he was living under a bridge and could not wait to see the look on his face when he moved into his home. First, though, I had to talk to the holistic doctor. There were cars on either side of mine. No one was even in them, but I felt so private about my situation that I kept the windows rolled up, so no one would hear my conversation. I don't know why. I acted like I had this terrible secret that I couldn't seem to let out, as if it was not just my genes but *I* that was defective.

I told the doctor about my BRCA status and explained that I was exploring my options. I said I was seriously considering having a hysterectomy and bilateral salpingo-oophorectomy but that I was worried about whether I'd be able to take hormones. This doctor told me I should not have the surgeries. She said there was "another way" to reduce my cancer risk. I wished I could believe that but something about her rubbed me the wrong way. She seemed way too sure that I had been receiving the wrong advice. In her medical practice, she focused on nutrition and balancing hormones. She would help me to a "point of health" where cancer cells would not develop. After what I'd learned about my faulty gene, I wasn't so sure. That night, I wrote in a journal I was keeping on BRCA appointments: "I don't think she understands BRCA issues or she wouldn't say that or shouldn't say that. I may have wasted $."

I wanted to believe in the "natural health," holistic approach. It would be great if eating the right diet and taking the right supplements could guarantee I would not get cancer. The fact that a poor diet can increase a person's cancer risk has been well-documented. But can a healthy diet loaded with fruits and vegetables ward off cancer in people with BRCA mutations? According to FORCE, there's not enough evidence yet to show whether and to what extent diet can help people with BRCA mutations.[7]

One of my doctor heroes, Dr. Dean Ornish, *Founder and President of the non-profit Preventive Medicine Research Institute and Clinical Professor of Medicine at the University of California, San Francisco,* inspired me to shoot for (not that I always succeed) a low-fat, plant-based diet long before I learned about my BRCA mutation. Ornish wrote in *Time* magazine that prophylactic surgery is a rational choice and that a healthy diet also can protect people with BRCA mutations. "Not everyone who eats meat, smokes, and is overweight, stressed, and sedentary gets breast cancer—protective genes may play a role. And you may eat well, move more, love well, and stress less and still die of breast cancer. Genes may override the best lifestyle, but not always," he said.[8] "While there is no assurance that lifestyle changes may prevent breast cancer in those who have the BRCA mutation, there is evidence that lifestyle changes are worth making, whether or not a person decides to undergo prophylactic surgery."

After all my complaining about the lack of clear guidance regarding the difficult choices that a BRCA mutation brings, I was more upset with a doctor telling me not to have surgery to reduce my risk. The holistic doctor said the next step would be an office visit. I said I needed to think about it. We hung up. I never contacted her again.

As I tried to figure out what to do, the most helpful resource of all was the nonprofit organization FORCE. Its focus on "facing our risk" was important because my first instinct was to run screaming in the opposite direction.

FORCE was started by Sue Friedman, a veterinarian who was diagnosed with breast cancer at age 33. After her treatment, she tested positive for a BRCA2 mutation. She founded FORCE in 1999 to provide much needed information to others at a time when little was available.

I spent countless hours on FORCE's website and message boards, reading stories of courageous women who had undergone or were considering undergoing double mastectomies and others who were choosing close surveillance instead. The site welcomes you into the world of "previvors"—those of us who face a high hereditary risk and have not been diagnosed with cancer. Inside that space, it's perfectly normal to have The Surgery. Or not. The tone was positive, matter of fact, and supportive. The message board has its own vocabulary and, thankfully, a glossary. PBM for prophylactic or preventative bilateral mastectomies. BC for breast cancer. Foobs for fake boobs. Ooph or BSO for bilateral salpingo-oophorectomy. The message boards were full of stories of fear, anxiety, indecision and encouragement. Breasts, for some, were "ticking time bombs." For those who were going to have PBMs, there were "ta ta to the ta tas" parties and recommendations for comfortable post-surgery loungewear and wipes to get you through the several days that you will not be allowed to shower. There were long discussions about various types of reconstruction and reports from women who traveled to some of the better-known facilities to have those doctors perform their surgeries. For those recovering from surgery, there were questions about pain, infections and rippling implants and gratitude for relief and peace of mind. It was a community of women who were willing to share their fears and answer each other's questions and offer comfort. Some of the screen names became so familiar, you felt like you knew the women. These women were smart and had done their homework.

For those unsure about whether they needed a PBM, some posted an analogy: "Would you get on an airplane that had an 85 percent chance of crashing?" Some looked on the bright side of PBMs and talked about how they'd have "perky" "foobs" into old age. Some were happy to go bigger than they had been. Some even got "tummy tucks" as part of the deal, with surgeons taking tissue from their stomachs to create new breasts. There were also posts about complications, pain, numbness and permanent loss of any sensation in their breasts, about husbands who were supportive and husbands who weren't. Overall, the takeaway was that the women who had gone through The Surgery felt that it was worth it because they had gained a lot of peace of mind. The sad images in my mind of women who had undergone PBMs changed as I realized how brave these women were for taking control of their health and making such a difficult decision.

On March 18, 2009, I nervously posted my own question on the FORCE message board:

> *I recently found out I'm BRCA2+ and cannot figure out what to do. I am trying to understand why many choose pbm (prophylactic bilateral mastectomy) over surveillance. What are the chances that surveillance will miss bc or find it in a late stage? Does this happen often and is that the main case for pbm? Thanks to anyone who can help.*

I got my first response 22 minutes later, followed my several other helpful comments for which I am so grateful:

A: Hi Kim, welcome to Force, where you will find plenty of support—and opinions! I am also BRCA2, found out this past November and have already had my ovaries and tubes out, as well as PBM, so I can surely understand the basis of your questions . . . Many women do also opt for surveillance, you'll see that, but I think it's a lot about risk tolerance and personal experience. For me, I have a very low risk tolerance when it comes to cancer; and for personal experience, I watched my mom whom I adored die of inflammatory BC, which is very aggressive and despite yearly mammos and annual visits to a breast surgeon, was found in Stage IV— liver and bones, mets to brain a year later, all bad. It just came on that quickly. When you've seen something like that, you want to avoid it for yourself.

Guest: I was dx with bc at the same time as I had genetic testing that told I was BRCA2. My mother had died of the disease as well as several of her first cousins. I opted for surveillance, feeling that with regular check ups, I was in good hands. However, after only 3½ years I have been dx with bc again—in my other breast and 2 weeks ago had BM. Now I have to have chemo again. Mammogram, ultrasound and physical exam did not identify bc. They found it when a lymph node popped up and biopsied positive for bc. Surveillance did not work for me. I had the PSO 3½ years ago.

R: I think you get to a point when surveillance just becomes too nerve-wracking . . . I'm BRCA2 but I'm also 53, when I read about the young women here having prophylactic mastectomies, I think they are the real heroes.

Me: thanks for all your responses. It's very scary to think that surveillance may not catch bc at an early stage. And I can relate to it getting too nerve wracking after having repeated *mammos, sonos, mris and four biopsies (benign) so far. I'm trying to get my mind around having a pbm but it's hard. And the few people I mention it to act like I'm overreacting by considering it. They haven't been through this though.*

AM: *I just found out I'm BRCA2+ last week. I'm for sure going to have PSO and probably hyst as soon as possible. I haven't got my head wrapped around the PBM either. I've known I was high risk for years but that test result last week brought me to this website and after reading and reading, the door has cracked open to considering BM. But I'm still not there yet . . . I think for now I'll keep researching and reading and try to keep the emotions in check.*

CC: *I was diagnosed with BRCA2 recently, too. I'm 34, have 2 kids, my mom survived metastatic breast cancer plus recurrence. After discussions with 6 or so different doctors and reading lots of academic papers, I'm going with prophylactic mastectomies and hysterectomy/bilateral salpingo-oophorectomy (uterine cancer in my family, too). But the decision wasn't easy, and I'm still debating timing—I think I'm going to do the mastectomy first and ooph before 40, but ask me tomorrow!! My reason for choosing surgeries are multifold, but come down to the fact that they are sure-fire ways of reducing your risk dramatically, and I don't think I could take the constant anxiety of surveillance alone. Anyway, it's a tough decision and your age, childbearing status, etc. will play into your decision, but know that you're not alone. I got a lot of "isn't that too drastic?" from a lot of the non-medical community, too, but I think given the statistics and the lack of options for us, it's not particularly drastic, it's just proactive. One poster once said, if you knew a plane had an 85 percent chance of crashing, would it be too drastic to cancel the flight? That really struck a chord with me.*

K: I found out in Nov. I had BRCA2. Even though when I went to test I knew I'd probably plan a pbm, when I actually got the results I stopped in my tracks. My head swam for two months . . . I was very stressed out initially.

I had a biopsy last year, which was painful and nerve-wracking. I had a hard time imagining going in twice a year for surveillance; even if they find cancer early, the thought of chemo terrifies me.

One of the things that helped me the most was reading on this board, and attending a local force meeting. Hearing so many stories of women who had surgery, and better yet, meeting them in person . . . they impressed me as strong, beautiful, athletic. Prior to my sister getting diagnosed with cancer last summer, I had never met anyone (that I knew of anyways) who had a mastectomy. My genetic counselor gave me a couple of names of local women who were willing to talk to me, a friend of mine gave me a contact as well. I think with each and every conversation, I became more comfortable with the idea of surgery, but it definitely took time. I am scheduled for April, and finally have a sense of peace and calm about my decision and what lies ahead. Give yourself time to do research, time to be sad, and hopefully you'll find a sense of what's right for you.

Sue Friedman posted: Welcome to FORCE and so sorry that you have cause to be here! . . . No matter where you are in the hereditary cancer spectrum and the decision-making spectrum there is nothing like our annual Joining FORCEs Conference to help you learn all you need to know to make informed decisions. This is the only conference by-and-for the hereditary cancer and BRCA community and I guarantee you will get a lot out of it.

I clicked the link to the conference, which was only a couple months away, scheduled in May, in Orlando.

I decided to go.

In May 2009, four months after I received my BRCA test results, I traveled to Orlando, Florida, for FORCE's national conference at the Buena Vista Palace Hotel & Spa. With sessions on hereditary cancer research, managing menopause, genetics, breast reconstruction and more, the three-day conference was a crash-course in all things BRCA. The conference featured sessions with some of the top BRCA researchers and other experts. There also was a "Show and Tell," where you could talk to women who'd had mastectomies about their surgeries and see the "results." One of the speakers was the prominent breast surgeon Dr. Susan Love, founder of the Dr. Susan Love Research Foundation. She was scheduled to give a session called "Breast Cancer Prevention: Nonsurgical Approach to Risk Reduction."

I flew to the conference by myself. I prefer to do things like this on my own. I need time alone to think and sort things out.

My husband encouraged me to go while he stayed home with our son. I'd been talking to him about what I'd discovered at my various appointments and in my research. We were both extremely confused about the whole thing. He encouraged my efforts to get the information I needed.

"I support you in whatever you decide," he said. At the same time, he said the idea of a double mastectomy was startling to him. He had some of the same concerns I had about whether surgery was the best option.

"Part of me wondered if maybe it wasn't too proactive for a cancer that might not even occur. Another part of me wondered what if the research at that time wasn't totally right—that maybe checkups and other preventative measures might be every bit as valuable as surgery, that perhaps some scientists were jumping the gun in suggesting surgery was the best option," he said when I recently asked him for his thoughts.

The trip would cost a lot: there was airfare, hotel and transportation to and from the hotel. We decided that it would be well worth the expense if it could help me better understand my options. I was nervous. Three days at a conference focused on breast cancer and ovarian cancer sounded depressing. I remember riding in a shuttle to the hotel with a friendly young couple headed to Disneyworld. They didn't have kids yet and were going for a fun vacation. It was a warm sunny spring day. There wasn't a cloud in the sky.

"What are you in Orlando for?" the guy asked in an eager voice. I'm sure Disneyworld is always the expected response in a cab ride from the Orlando airport.

"I'm here for a conference," I said, smiling.

"Oh, what's the conference?" he asked in a friendly tone.

I didn't mention the type of conference before to avoid being a Debbie Downer in the Happiest Place on Earth. These nice people didn't need to hear about the big C. What could I do? He asked.

"It's called FORCE. It's a conference for people with a hereditary risk of breast cancer," I said, trying to make it sound as positive as possible. I didn't want them to have to think about breast cancer on their vacation.

"Oh," they both said and made a comment about how it sounded like a helpful conference.

At the hotel, I found the registration table and checked in. I got a big binder with a schedule and information on speakers and presentations.

"Be sure to get your beads," the woman at the table said.

Next to it was a table full of colorful bead necklaces. There was purple for those of us who were high-risk but had never been diagnosed with cancer (called previvors). Pink for breast cancer survivors. Teal for ovarian cancer survivors. Orange for BRCA1 mutations. Dark Blue for BRCA2 mutations. Dark green for those who hadn't had testing. And other colors for healthcare providers and supporters/spouses/partners. I chose the color for BRCA2 and for previvor. FORCE coined the term in 2000 and it has become widely used since then. The conference started with a welcome from Sue Friedman and other speakers. Next, I went to a session called "Genetics 101."

That afternoon, I attended a session titled "Making Decisions about Your Cancer Risk," led by Dr. Karen Hurley, a psychologist who specializes in hereditary cancer risk. *Hurley talked about three stages of the decision-making process. First, there's the* cognitive level that includes collecting and understanding the facts. Second is the emotional level of dealing with feelings about the decision and how it fits into other parts of life including family and life plans. The third is the post-decision level, in which you have the knowledge, coping strategies and support to carry out the decision. I was definitely stuck in the first stage.

Hurley also talked about how frustrating and uncomfortable the state of uncertainty can be while you're going through the decision-making process. She emphasized that we need to be able to tolerate that discomfort until we fully explore the issue. This requires trusting that once you complete the process, the decision will "gel" into place. I wrote in my notes not to "rush into a decision because of the discomfort of uncertainty." On the other hand, endless researching can be a delay tactic, she said.

Decisions about whether to have surgery require you to accept that none of the choices is ideal and that future advances may make today's choices look primitive. Hurley emphasized that everyone is different about how much information they want to seek out about a health threat. She talked about how too much information can heighten anxiety for some by keeping them focused on the threat.

At the sessions, I saw people who—based on their bead colors—like me had not been diagnosed with cancer. We were there to figure out how to prevent our worst nightmare. Others were already dealing with it. I can't forget a young woman, probably still in her 20s, who was pale, thin and frail-looking. She wore a beautiful floral scarf over her head. I couldn't imagine how hard it must be to go through a cancer diagnosis at an age when you're just starting your adult life. A BRCA mutation diagnosis can be especially difficult for younger women who still want to have children. It puts even greater pressure on the biological clock.

At lunch, I just found a table and sat down next a mother and daughter from southern California. The daughter was in her 20s and had a BRCA mutation. They wore the same color of beads, for BRCA2 mutations. We talked over salads and iced tea about how we had recently discovered our BRCA statuses and how we did not know what to do.

One of the most helpful parts of the conference was the "Birds of a Feather Show and Tell" event. That's where, on Friday and Saturday nights of the conference, women who have had mastectomies share their stories and show what their reconstructed breasts look like. Plastic surgeons were also there to answer any questions. There was wine and cheese. It almost felt like a party. I was nervous as I walked up a stairway to the "Show and Tell" room.

I was expecting that the women who were doing the "showing" would take visitors to a dressing area and lift their shirt to show their surgery results. I felt silly for thinking that once I got to the room, however. There were several women without tops on and they were standing around, sipping wine and talking casually to small groups of women as if they were chatting about a new movie rather than mastectomies and reconstruction. Most of them had reconstruction after their mastectomies, though I saw one woman who had "gone flat." She had long scars across her chest from her mastectomies. I had a lot of respect for her decision and for her courage to participate in the event. When I saw her, though, I quickly looked away. Seeing her scars was jarring, much more so than seeing women who had beautifully reconstructed breasts to show off. The scars on the woman who did not go through reconstruction forced me to see what is lost in a mastectomy. The perfect foobs the other women had made The Surgery seem like less of a loss to me.

I stood by the entry as if I was afraid to go in. I felt awkward. I looked around. It was a nice room with comfy chairs. I started talking to a woman standing near the door. She was pretty, probably around 30. She had perfect-looking breasts, probably C cups. You couldn't even see her scars. I wanted those.

I said hi, still feeling awkward standing there, in my jeans and T-shirt, chatting with this woman who wasn't wearing a shirt. I asked her about her surgery.

"You look great," I said.

"Thanks. I'm so happy with my results."

"When did you have your surgery?"

"Last year."

"Did you get saline or silicone implants?"

"Silicone."

I avoided looking directly at her breasts until she showed me her scars. If she hadn't pointed them out, I wouldn't have seen them. They were under her breast, along the bottom. I had never seen the results of a breast reconstruction surgery up close. It was truly amazing. They did not have the fake stripper boob look that I was somehow expecting.

I didn't stay long. Show and Tell was a great program. It was weird though. I still could not even say the M word.

The information at the FORCE conference was a lot to take in. I was overwhelmed at the prospect of surgeries, surveillance and worrying about cancer. Because I didn't have cancer, I tried to avoid feeling sad about the whole thing, as if I didn't have the right. It's not good, but I tend to keep my problems to myself. I hate to burden anyone. That's one of the reasons that the conference was so helpful: everyone understood what each other was going through.

In between sessions, I visited the exhibitors' area. It was another eye-opening experience. That's where I met the Robert Palmer girls. They reminded me of the models in the singer's music video because they were tall, thin, perfectly dressed and coiffed and were like backup singers to plastic surgeons who were known for their artistic work. Several of the plastic surgeons at the event had their own set of models who had undergone mastectomies at the surgeons' clinic. I flipped through a book of photos at their table showing the surgeon's "results." There were photos showing women's breasts, just the chest area of their bodies. They were stunning. One of the Robert Palmer girls asked me if I had any questions.

I told her that I was diagnosed with the BRCA2 mutation and didn't know what to do. She said she's a doctor and that she decided to get preventative surgery. She said she had saline implants. She said they were harder than silicone, but she didn't want silicone in her body.

That's one of the choices along the way that women must face—what type of implant to get: Silicone or saline. The pros and cons of each are an entire research project.

"I'm so happy with the results," she said.

"You look great," I said, nodding. I never thought I'd be telling a woman how great her breasts looked. But there I was. I asked her if she had experienced much pain through the process.

"It wasn't that bad at all," she said. "I was nervous, but I had very little pain."

One of the sessions I did not want to miss was the Breast Reconstruction Overview session featuring Kathy Steligo, author of *The Breast Reconstruction Handbook*. Steligo out-lined the various types of reconstruction procedures and gave practical advice about recovery times for each of the differ-ent surgeries. If you decide you want foobs, the next ques-tion is what kind? If you go with implants, you have to decide what kind. Saline ones are hard. Silicone feel more natural. If saline implants rupture, they'll just leak water into your body. I remember the lawsuits and women's complaints of health concerns that led to a ban on silicone implants from 1992 to 2006. I'd even interviewed a few women involved in one of the cases and heard first-hand her story of the pain her rup-tured implants had caused. How horrible would it be to put in a silicone implant that leaked and caused health problems? The FDA and all the plastic surgeons I talked to said silicone implants were safe now. They were made of a thicker gummy-bear-like substance that would not leak if the implants rup-tured. I hoped it was true.

Implants had some advantages over reconstruction using my own tissue, in my mind. Implants are a less intensive sur-gery with a faster recovery time than surgeries that transfer tissue from your stomach, butt or back to create new breasts. The tissue-transfer involves much larger incisions and a longer healing process. When the surgery is done, though, you're done. Implants typically involve a multi-step process, starting with expanders, which are temporary, and a second surgery to exchange those with implants. Some surgeons will put in the implants during the mastectomy surgery in what's called a "one-step" procedure. The plastic surgeons I spoke to, however, don't do one steps because they say they don't get the best results with the procedure. Another thing to remember is that implants don't last forever. They need to be replaced at some point, while tissue-transfer reconstruction is permanent. There are so many questions and considerations, it can drive you nuts.

I left to take a break in my room. I was on information overload. I still couldn't get my head around a double mastectomy and reconstruction. But I was encouraged about The Surgery after talking to several women at the conference. The ones who had gotten double mastectomies were at peace with their decisions. I wanted some of that.

"I have anxiety. I don't do well with uncertainty," one woman I met said. "My surgery gave me peace of mind."

Having the surgery to gain peace of mind made sense to me. If you have the mastectomies, and the bilateral salpingo-oophorectomy, I figured you can know that you've done everything in your power to reduce your risk of cancer. You can still get cancer, though the risk is low. What else can you do? I thought of my mom asking her mom, my grandmother, why she didn't see a doctor for months after feeling a lump in her breast. It was painful to think about that conversation. I could only imagine how hard that was for each of them. If I was diagnosed with breast cancer, I did not want to face any regrets that I had not been more proactive. I couldn't stand the idea of Leo asking and having to wonder why I hadn't done what I could to prevent my illness.

That fall, my mom and I attended a one-day conference hosted by genetic counselors in Dallas. It was held at a cancer support center called Gilda's Club, in honor of Gilda Radner, who died of ovarian cancer at age 42—my age at the time. (The name of the club later changed and is now Cancer Support Community.) Some have speculated that Radner probably had a BRCA mutation because she was so young and had a family history of cancer. Radner wrote in her book, *It's Always Something*,[9] about the support she received at the Wellness Center, a similar place in Santa Monica. Gilda's Club and the Wellness Center merged in 2009 to become the Cancer Support Community. I grew up seeing Radner and her characters on *Saturday Night Live*. Radner's husband, Gene Wilder, said she wanted to give back to the program so that other people living with cancer would have the type of emotional support she received. At one point, I was walking down the hall to find a bathroom. I saw a photo of Radner, beautiful and smiling, and teared up. Radner, who was such a brilliant comedian and could find humor in just about anything, called cancer "probably the most unfunny thing in the world."

Back in the conference, there were about 40 of us sitting in rows of folding chairs listening to a panel of three or four women, one in her 20s, who were talking about their experiences of having double mastectomies. I was impressed. They seemed so smart and brave. They were upbeat, smart, stylish and attractive, not the sad, anxiety-ridden, sick-looking people that somehow previously had inhabited the images in my head. These women were happy and confident about their choices. They felt like they had taken charge of their lives and could reassure themselves they had done all they could to prevent cancer. I wanted to be like them when I grow up.

The panelists talked about different types of breast reconstruction. I learned that having mastectomies means you probably will lose all sensation in your breasts. One of the women said she recovered some feeling. The women recommended talking to more than one plastic surgeon. They emphasized that mastectomies have changed since the days of the radical mastectomy that were the standard of care until the 1970s. A plastic surgeon discussed the procedure and showed headless photos of reconstructed breasts that blew me away. The surgeon's "results" were gorgeous. I realized that for me, this surgery could be a major upgrade. Mastectomies still sounded horrible, but a little less awful than I initially imagined.

One of the women on the panel made a point that I had not considered.

"I'd rather tackle this while I'm healthy," she said. I heard that again later in my research. Reconstruction can be much more complicated after cancer radiation, for example.

Another quote I jotted down made an important point about the advantage of preventing, rather than surviving cancer.

"Our situation is about living, not just survival," she said.

Some of the panelists decided to get the surgery soon after finding out they had BRCA mutations; others took time to make their choice.

"When you're ready, you'll know you're ready," one of the women said.

Each of them said the best benefit was a feeling of relief.

"If I got cancer, wouldn't you want to know you did everything you could to prevent it?" one of them said.

A breast surgeon spoke about the latest treatments for breast cancer and promising new treatments on the horizon. Afterward, I approached her with a question that I still couldn't shake. I told her I have a BRCA2 mutation and that I was worried about surveillance.

"How much of a chance is there that mammograms and MRIs would miss a cancer?" I asked.

"They should catch it," she said reassuringly, as if there wasn't much to worry about. That word—*should*—really bothered me.

One of the best things about the FORCE message boards was meeting Bonnie, the first person I met outside my family who had a BRCA mutation. Bonnie had posted something asking about women's experiences with doctors in Dallas. She wanted to get in touch with other Dallas women and posted her email. I decided to write. We traded a few emails and realized we had a lot in common. Both of us had recently learned we had BRCA2 mutations and neither of us knew what to do. She lived in Dallas and was close to my age. We traded a few emails then decided to meet for lunch at an Italian restaurant. I was nervous—I'd only met her online—but we hit it off immediately. It was wonderful to have someone to talk to who was going through the exact same thing. She had done a ton of research. Although I had talked to my husband, mom and sisters about BRCA, I needed support from someone who was in the same point of their decision-making process.

By this time, I had a growing list of pros and cons of having a prophylactic bilateral mastectomy. I had the luxury of time—and the fear that I was taking too much of it. I desperately searched for ammunition for the "cons" side of my list, but kept finding more "pros:"

- I want to be proactive.
- It's better to prevent, rather than wait for, cancer.
- Surveillance may not catch cancer early.

- Mastectomies are more difficult after a cancer diagnosis, with issues such as radiated skin.
- Surveillance every six months, and the biopsies that follow, are very stressful.
- Feeling of relief that you've done all you can.
- Some doctors strongly recommend mastectomies (while others say surveillance is fine).
- Risk would be less than that of the general population.
- There are some cancers that are aggressive and could grow fast between screenings.
- Some cancers don't show up on mammograms or MRIs.
- BRCA2 breast cancer risk increases dramatically at age 40.
- Would regret not having surgery if develop cancer.
- Want to do the best thing possible to reduce risk and be able to be a mother to Leo as long as possible.
- BC is the #1 cause of death in women in my age group. BC is often found later and more aggressive at my age.
- I feel like I am gambling without the surgery.
- Breast cancer sucks and it can kill you.

CHAPTER 4

Pinkwashed

"Let me die of anything but suffocation by the pink sticky sentiment embodied in that teddy bear."

—Barbara Ehrenreich, breast cancer survivor and writer[1]

The more I learned, the more I felt like my understanding of breast cancer had been pinkwashed. I knew breast cancer was serious—it killed my grandmother and great-grandmother. However, most of the news I'd seen about breast cancer focused on feel-good stories about breast cancer survivors who were thriving thanks to early detection. The message I took in was that mammograms would catch any breast cancer early, I'd get treatment, and be okay. I started to realize that, while this may be mostly true, it's not always true. I had no idea that mammograms may miss as many as 20 percent of cancers, especially in younger women, who typically have denser breast tissue that makes cancer more difficult to detect (and BRCA-related cancers typically strike women at younger ages).[2] I didn't realize that even Stage 1 breast cancer can kill you. Or that some tumors are aggressive and can grow and become invasive between annual mammograms. Or that some breast cancer cells can enter the bloodstream and spread to other parts of the body—even in early-stage cancers.

I felt like I'd been viewing the whole thing through pink-colored glasses. In the upbeat hopeful narrative that has focused on the wonderful and real possibility of survivorship, women are painted as brave warriors and we celebrate their victories in the battle against cancer. We rarely hear about women, who are just as courageous, who lose the fight against the horrible disease. The reality is that breast cancer kills about 40,000 women in the United States[3] and 522,000 women worldwide each year.[4]

Breast cancer is the second-leading cause of cancer deaths among women, behind lung cancer, in the United States, according to the nonprofit breastcancer.org.[5] There has been a lot of progress in the search for a cure and a lot of frustration that so many women are still dying of the disease. In 2018, there were 266,120 expected cases of invasive breast cancer in the United States.[6] Another 63,960 women each year are diagnosed with non-invasive breast cancer, sometimes called Stage 0 breast cancer. The most common type of non-invasive breast cancer is ductal carcinoma in situ, or DCIS. DCIS can become invasive; however, the abnormal cells may never spread beyond the milk ducts.[7]

The more I learned, the more I worried about having breast cancer at *any* stage.

My anxiety zeroed in on the fact that screenings can miss some cancers. This was a huge issue to me. If I couldn't rely on screenings to catch breast cancer at an early, treatable stage, that might be a deal breaker. The odds are that mammograms and MRIs will identify cancers at early stages, but I never realized or thought about the fact that they are no guarantee. After one of my mammograms, which came back showing no suspicious areas, I received a letter from the mammography center that included a sobering statement: "Although Mammography is an excellent diagnostic tool, it is not infallible. Please remember that mammography does not detect approximately 10–15 percent of breast cancers. We encourage you to follow the American Cancer Society guidelines for the early detection of breast cancer. These guidelines include monthly breast self-examination, annual physical examination by a health care professional, and annual screening mammography after the age of 40." I could not stop reading the line: "Mammography does not detect approximately 10–15 percent of breast cancers."

I became increasingly concerned about screenings and the fact that cancers that are caught early can become fatal. I thought that these were two of the most important issues in deciding about whether to have risk-reducing double mastectomy. I posted a question about it on the FORCE message board:

Chance of metastasis with early stage BC [breast cancer]? 10/26/2010

Does anyone know the chance of a distant recurrence if you're diagnosed with early stage BC? I am BRCA2+ and struggling with the decision of whether to have a PBM. I am wondering if I continue with surveillance and am diagnosed with Stage 1 cancer, what would be the chance of having a distant metastasis? I have been told that if you catch BC early, you'll be treated and you'll be OK. But is that a false sense of security? I worry what are the chances it could spread? And what are the chances that the cancer won't be caught early in the first place?

The answers shattered my illusions about early-stage breast cancer.

Guest: *I struggled with these exact same questions when I was at your stage and I posed these questions to my doctors, who I would say were neutral or even more in favor of surveillance. Though the odds are in your favor and are changing as treatment and detection improves, they still weren't willing to put numbers on this and would only keep saying, "There are no guarantees."*

In the meantime, I've heard enough anecdotes on here and from acquaintances that tell of how cancers either went undetected or developed and grew between screenings, or how radiation treatment for early stage cancer caused a second cancer, etc. that I'm so glad I went for the PBM (prophylactic bilateral mastectomy). I have a low personal tolerance for risk and so even if they had put a number on it, say 95 percent, I couldn't have handled the anxiety with that leftover 5 percent. As a BRCA2+ person, I feel like I have enough leftover risk for other cancers even after PBM and ooph. I am glad this was one I could minimize.

Guest: *There is not one specific risk number for distant metastasis associated with early bc (breast cancer). It is a crap shoot. For me that is part of the issue. Even if the tumor is caught "early" you can't predict beforehand what the pathology will be. A tumor that turns out to be a small, well differentiated, low grade, very slow growing, highly er/pr positive her2 negative tumor will have a very different recurrence rate compared to a small, undifferentiated, rapidly growing, high grade, triple negative tumor. Also, even if you deal with a bc diagnosis and it is caught early and the pathology is "good," it is possible that years later you can have another primary tumor with a very different pathology.*

Guest: *The common thinking seems to be if you catch BC early it usually hasn't metastasized. However, with BRCA especially, I feel like all bets are off. My mom found it between screenings (didn't know her BRCA2 status) and right away it was aggressive and had metastasized. So the problem becomes, statistics are great when you're on the right side of them. But someone makes up that other percentage.*

Guest: *What tipped the scales for me 4 years ago: a consult with Dr. K when he told me that no matter what or how frequent* *my surveillance, he could not guarantee that breast cancer would be found in a curable stage.*

Guest: *Another thing to consider is the possibility of a 2nd primary bc diagnosis. I was told by my oncologist that there was a 50 percent chance of a second primary tumor in BRCA positive women.*

Another woman wrote back, quoting a woman who was a frequent poster on the site:

You don't want to catch this early, my friend. YOU DON'T WANT TO CATCH IT AT ALL.

The woman she was quoting had made a lot of friends on the message board and often shared her story and advice. If you followed the message board, you felt like you knew her. She had a BRCA1 mutation and was struggling with what is called triple negative breast cancer, an especially aggressive type. She died two months after that post. During her last days, women posted messages thanking her for answering questions and sharing her experiences and advice. I wished I could thank her for her post. That thread about catching BC early was so powerful. I couldn't get her comment out of my mind.

In the book, *Positive Results, Making the Best Decisions When You're at High Risk for Breast or Ovarian Cancer,* Joi L. Morris and co-authors wrote that doctors recommend breast imaging each six months, with alternating MRI and mammograms, beginning at an age at least 10 years younger than the earliest breast cancer onset in the family and no later than age 30 (and no earlier than 20). "While this combination of MRI with mammography has excellent potential to detect cancers very early, the detection rate will likely never reach 100 percent of tumors at a stage when they are curable. Because BRCA tumors are often highly aggressive, it is important to recognize that even a very small tumor, detected at what may seem to be an early stage, may be fatal. Maybe not in a large percentage of women, but certainly in some. For this reason, most experts advise women who do intend to pursue a plan of surveillance consider other risk-reduction measures such as bilateral salpingo-oophorectomy or chemoprevention."[8]

The words "even a small tumor, detected at what may seem to be an early stage, may be fatal." What? This was news to me. It was shocking. And it scared the hell out of me.

As I was weighing whether to have risk-reducing surgery, Elizabeth Edwards, who was married to then-presidential candidate John Edwards, was going through her highly publicized battle with metastatic breast cancer. Elizabeth Edwards, whose cancer was not caused by a BRCA mutation, initially was diagnosed with breast cancer in 2004 after discovering a large lump while on the campaign trail with her husband. In her book, *Resilience*,[9] Edwards wrote that bone and liver scans were clear at the time. She had chemotherapy and radiation. She recovered from her illness and was doing well until 2007, when she announced the cancer had spread but that she was hopeful. In 2010, the news got worse: Edwards was dying. She had been open about her illness, saying that she had not gotten mammograms as regularly as she should have. She urged women to take care of their health. Edwards was candid about the precariousness of her prognosis from the beginning, telling the program *Dateline* in 2004: "You know, there are no guarantees on prognosis. I mean, if you don't have metastasis, and we don't know that I don't. But we don't have any indication that I do. Then your prognosis is better. But there are no guarantees with this. Even if you get rid of it, is there some tiny cell someplace that's you know going to grow again. . . . You're not going to know it. But you know there are no guarantees in life anyway. And if the one thing that we've learned over the years is that you're going to have to live every day like it's your last day anyway. So you know, this, for me, it's just another reminder of that lesson."[10]

Edwards died in December 2010. She was 61. Her devastating cancer recurrence raised awareness about metastatic cancer, which does not get enough attention in the public discussion about breast cancer. In 2013, Edwards' older daughter, Cate Edwards, quoted a startling—and disputed—statistic about metastatic breast cancer in a column on CNN's website: "Many of us don't realize that 20% to 30% of all breast cancer cases will become metastatic. I know this personally because I experienced it with my mom, Elizabeth, when she was diagnosed with metastatic breast cancer in 2007."[11]

That statistic, which comes from a 2005 research paper in the journal *The Oncologist*,[12] is the subject of debate. Regardless of what percentage of cancers become metastatic, the fact that some early-stage breast cancers become deadly points to a dark truth that gets overshadowed in the upbeat pink ribbon culture that dominates breast cancer awareness.

That fall, in 2010, I pitched a story to my editor about the increased use of genetic testing to identify women at high risk of breast cancer. I hadn't seen many articles about BRCA in the news and it was Breast Cancer Awareness Month. I didn't tell my boss that I had a personal interest in the subject. It was still too hard to talk about and I was afraid I would start crying if I mentioned it. For the story, I found a couple of women who had BRCA mutations and were willing to be interviewed. I met one of them, Carrie, at a Starbucks on a beautiful sunny October afternoon. Fall weather is gorgeous in Dallas, with a touch of coolness that comes as a relief after brutal triple-digit summers. We sat at a table on the patio as Carrie told me about how she had been diagnosed with Stage 2 breast cancer at age 29, just weeks before her wedding. She said she felt a lump that had appeared suddenly. She was too young to have to deal with cancer. Stage 2 means that the cancer is still contained in the breast or has only spread to nearby lymph nodes, according to the American Cancer Society. Stage 2 is considered early stage and comes with a good prognosis. Carrie did not realize she had a BRCA2 mutation until she was diagnosed. Hers had spread to the lymph nodes. She had a double mastectomy and several rounds of chemotherapy. She was beautiful, smart and upbeat and she did not sugarcoat her experience. Her dark brown hair had just started to grow back after chemotherapy.

I confided that I also had a BRCA2 mutation and that I was considering my options. She said she would have had a double mastectomy to prevent her risk if she had known she carried the BRCA mutation before she had cancer.

"What's holding you back?" she asked.

I paused. I didn't have a good answer. I wasn't even sure. She recommended her doctor, who she said held her hand to comfort her before her surgery. I met him in one of my numerous consultations. When I asked him what I should do, he had that somber look I'd seen in several of my doctors' eyes and said I should strongly consider The Surgery.

I ran into Carrie a year or so later at a nonprofit event I was covering for *The News*. She was doing PR for a company that was involved. She looked vibrant and appeared to be thriving. She asked me if I'd had my surgery. "Not yet." I said, adding that I was still trying to "get there." My hesitancy must have seemed to her like a waste of a precious gift of a warning. I kept thinking of her question about what was holding me back. I didn't have the insight at the time to be able to tell the truth: "Because I'm paralyzed by fear and anxiety."

I recently searched her name online to see how she was doing. I was hoping to find on LinkedIn that she had moved up in her career. I felt sick to my stomach when I found her obituary. I learned that Carrie was diagnosed with a Stage 4 recurrence in 2012, two years after I had met her. She wrote on a cancer blog in 2015 that her cancer had spread to her lungs, liver, bones and brain. She endured rounds of chemotherapy, radiation and other treatments. She died several months later, leaving behind the four-year-old son she and her husband had adopted before she learned that her cancer had returned. She was buried on her 36th birthday. Several months before she died, Carrie wrote in her blog, "The gold standard drugs have all failed me and now the doctors are asking me what I want to do next. I'm at the point in my treatment where I'm too educated to believe I can live with metastatic breast cancer for three decades like a chronic disease, but I'm still holding on to the hope of seeing a game-changing medical breakthrough in my lifetime."[13]

It was so heart-breaking. And so unfair.

I felt like over the years, I'd received overly positive messages about breast cancer. It feels good to hear stories about women who "beat" breast cancer and that early detection saves lives. We need hope. But have we been getting an overly optimistic picture? It felt like I'd been told a white lie—really, a pink lie—to make us all feel empowered to fight breast cancer. We see the beautiful smiling faces, the courageous warriors, the pink ribbons and messages such as "Fight Like a Girl" in the messages about breast cancer. We rarely hear about the also courageous women who die every day from the disease. I used to think that most of them, like my grandmother and great-grandmother, had unfortunately not been diagnosed or treated until it was too late. I had no idea that most of them had caught their cancers in earlier stages—but their cancers later progressed to Stage 4.

The bottom line is that no one can guarantee that screenings will catch breast cancer early. And no one can be sure that even if breast cancer is caught early, it will not become terminal.

Los Angeles Times reporter Laurie Becklund wrote shortly before she died of breast cancer in 2015 that her death was proof that early-stage cancers can kill. She wrote about how more than 20 mammograms missed her disease:[14]

> In 1996, during a self-exam, I found a peanut-sized lump in one breast that turned out to be Stage 1 breast cancer. I had the "best," most common, kind of breast cancer, found it early, and got a lumpectomy and short dose of radiation. Five years out, my doctor told me there was little chance of recurrence and said, "Have a great life!"
>
> You can imagine my shock when, 13 years after my initial diagnosis, I was in gridlock on the Harbor Freeway and got a call from my doctor with the results of a PET scan ordered after routine blood labs. "Maybe you should pull over," he said.

There's plenty of anecdotal evidence of screenings that missed cancers and early stage cancers that morphed into deadly ones. I wanted statistics. How many cases of early stage cancer end up metastasizing? How can this be happening when I've heard all my adult life that mammograms and early detection were the key to staying healthy? And why aren't people talking—and getting more concerned—about it? I spent countless hours researching, looking for answers that didn't seem to exist.

Metastatic breast cancer means that the cancer started in the breast and spread to another part of the body, according to the National Cancer Institute. Only about 6 percent of breast cancers are diagnosed after they have become metastatic, called Stage 4. That means most women who die of breast cancer had tumors that initially were diagnosed at earlier stages and later metastasized despite treatment.

A 2017 study on metastatic breast cancer (MBC) in the journal *Cancer Epidemiology, Biomarkers & Prevention* estimated that 138,622 women in the United States were living with metastatic breast cancer in 2013, the most recent data available.[15] Of those women, 38,897—28 percent—were initially diagnosed at Stage 4.[16] Most of them, 99,725, were initially diagnosed with earlier stages of breast cancer that progressed to Stage 4.[17]

"This study demonstrates a growing burden of MBC in the United States. It also makes clear that the majority of patients with MBC, the three out of four who are diagnosed with non-metastatic cancer but progress to distant disease, has never been properly documented. Given the growing burden of MBC, it is critical to collect data on recurrence to foster more research into the specific needs of this understudied population," the authors wrote in the study funded by the National Institute of Health.[18]

The fact that early cancers can spread goes against what I once believed about breast cancer. We typically think of breast cancer starting with a small tumor that grows and can get into the lymph nodes and then spread to other parts of the body. The path, however, is not always that clear-cut. The science is still unfolding. Breastcancer.org, a nonprofit organization dedicated to providing the most reliable, complete, and up-to-date information about breast cancer, explains on its web page about metastatic cancer that: "When you had surgery to remove the original breast cancer, your surgeon removed all the cancer that could be seen and felt. But tests for cancer aren't sensitive enough to detect a tiny group of single cancer cells. These isolated cells may survive radiation therapy and chemotherapy aimed at preventing recurrence. Even a single cell that escaped treatment may be able to spread and grow into a tumor."[19]

Only a fraction of breast cancer research funding and seemingly little media coverage on the topic focuses on metastasis. Advocates in the metastatic breast cancer community point out that the story of hope and success creates a better narrative for fundraising campaigns.

"Non-metastatic patients are frightened by us and our condition. They don't like hearing that 30 percent of them will go on to metastasize and that it can happen now or as many as 35 years into the future despite healthy lifestyles, excellent medical care and early detection," said CJ Corneliussen-James, Director Emeritus and Founder of the national non-profit, METAvivor Research and Support (metavivor.org) and an MBC patient, who provided an interview for this book. METAvivor has funded $4.2 million in MBC research grants, established over 60 MBC peer support programs and runs a national Stage 4 cancer advocacy program.

Decades ago, breast cancer awareness campaigns took the disease from something no one would mention to something everyone knows about. I have worn pink ribbon T-shirts and had coffee out of pink mugs and love the color pink. Somewhere along the line, though, we moved from awareness to putting such a rosy tint on the picture of breast cancer that some of us are overly optimistic about our risk. Maybe we need fewer pink ribbons on buckets of unhealthy fried chicken, fewer "save the boobies" wristbands and fewer pink ribbon stuffed animals that infantilize breast cancer, as writer Barbara Ehrenreich wrote in her "Welcome to Cancerland" essay. (As Ehrenreich said, "certainly we don't give Matchbox cars to men with prostate cancer.")[20]

As I tried to decide what to do, that post on the FORCE board kept haunting me: "You don't want to catch this early, my friend. YOU DON'T WANT TO CATCH IT AT ALL."

Until my BRCA diagnosis, I had never had to consider the fact, even if you survive cancer, your life will never be quite the same. You may need radiation and/or chemo and tamoxifen, even for Stage 1 cancer, that has lasting effects such as fertility concerns if you want to have children, not to mention the hell of chemo itself, and constant fear about whether any cancer cells have spread to other parts of your body or whether the cancer could "come back." Surveillance should work for most women. But it started to feel like too much of a gamble. I'd found plenty of evidence that made me seriously consider The Surgery.

The bottom line for me became: What would give me the best chance of living a healthy life for as long as possible—a risk-reducing mastectomy or close surveillance? I expected the answer to be a double mastectomy. I shouldn't have been surprised that the answer was as murky and complicated as everything else regarding BRCA. It's a tossup according to the limited amount of research on the topic. Here was one more confusing piece of information to muddy the path to a decision: A 2010 *Journal of Clinical Oncology* study found that women with BRCA mutations who had risk-reducing mastectomies and risk-reducing oophorectomies—did not have a significantly greater chance of living longer than women who only had their ovaries removed.[21]

The lead author of the study, Dr. Allison Kurian, associate professor of medicine (oncology) and of Health Research and Policy and Director of Women's Clinical Cancer Genetics Program at Stanford University School of Medicine, said she hoped the study could help women in their decision-making.

"I certainly don't have any 'right answers' when it comes to these very challenging decisions, and I have not had to make them myself, so I will never truly know what it feels like. However, I've had the privilege of working with high-risk women for the last 15 years, and I have great respect for the courage and thoughtfulness with which women deliberate these hard choices. My colleagues and I built the decision tool in the hope that it might help women to visualize and compare their options more clearly, and thus make these difficult decisions a little bit easier. I have observed that most women ultimately find the path that feels right to them—whether it be intensive screening or prophylactic surgery—and that most seem to be at peace with the choices they have made," Kurian said.[22]

The table below reports estimated survival to age 70 for several groups of simulated BRCA carriers.

Survival to Age 70	Survival %
General population	84
BRCA1	
No intervention	53
Surveillance, no surgical intervention	59
Surveillance, oophorectomy at age 40	74
PBM at 40,* oophorectomy at age 40	77
PBM at 25, oophorectomy at age 40	79
BRCA2	
No intervention	71
Surveillance, no surgical intervention	75
Surveillance, oophorectomy at age 50	79
Surveillance, oophorectomy at age 40	80
PBM at 25, oophorectomy at age 40	83
PBM at 40,* oophorectomy at age 50	83

SOURCE: {Kurian, 2010, Survival Analysis of Cancer Risk Reduction Strategies for BRCA1/2 Mutation}

More research will be needed on long-term survival of women who get The Surgery. A study in the *American Journal of Surgery* documented a need for longer follow-up to more data to determine the survival benefit from risk-reducing mastectomies.[23] Studies so far have relied on small samples and short follow-up periods.

"The reduction in breast cancer risk with BRRM (breast risk-reducing mastectomy), however, has not translated into a survival benefit in primary studies, likely because of short-term follow-up," the researchers found. "BRRM may eventually demonstrate a significant survival advantage given the reduction in breast cancer incidence as longer follow-up of these mutation carriers becomes available."[24]

Even if time does not show that women who have risk-reducing surgery live longer, survival simply means that the person is alive. It does not measure quality of life, including the toll that radiation and chemotherapy take on a person. It's impossible to quantify the benefits of enjoying good health vs. surviving cancer treatments and worrying that cancer will return. You might live to 70 either way, but life after a cancer diagnosis will never be the same. That leads some women with BRCA mutations to decide that if they're probably going to need to have a double mastectomy eventually, they may as well do it before they will also need chemotherapy and/or radiation.

CHAPTER 5

False Alarms

"Living with BRCA, every time I have a pain in my breast, or I have any kind of feeling of being bloated, or just a fear, it's constantly in the back of my mind: am I going to get cancer? When am I going to get cancer? Am I going to be able to fight it? Once you know that predisposition is there, it's very hard not to think about yourself as someone who will eventually get these diseases if you don't do something about it. So you are constantly looking over your shoulder and pleading not to get these diseases."[1]

—Joanna Rudnick, BRCA1 mutation carrier, breast cancer survivor, filmmaker, *In the Family*

While I tried to figure out what to do, I ended up choosing surveillance by default.

Surveillance means you get screened every six months. For me, it was a mammogram in January and an MRI in June. In between, my doctors did clinical breast exams, which meant I had some type of check every few months. Surveillance had its advantages: I didn't have to go through surgery and I knew that my screenings probably would catch any problems early.

It sounded easy enough, much easier than having surgery. I imagined that I'd go in for my mammogram or MRI and that I wouldn't have to worry about it until the next screening time six months later, kind of like getting an oil change. I wasn't prepared for the fact that the tests can mean multiple appointments, lunch breaks spent at the doctor, costly co-pays and lots of worry. MRIs are expensive, especially if you have crappy insurance. One year, I had a high-deductible plan that forced me to pay $1,800 for the test. It took me a year and a half of monthly $200 payments—money I didn't have to begin with—to pay it off. Just in time for the next screening. Thankfully, by that time I had better insurance.

The worst part—aside from the fact that there was no guarantee surveillance would detect cancer early—was the false alarms. Mammograms can highlight areas that may be problematic or that may be nothing at all. MRIs can raise red flags about "suspicious" areas that also turn out to be benign. Radiologists can't always tell whether an area that lights up the screen is something or nothing. The only way to tell sometimes is to do a biopsy. False alarms are part of the bargain with surveillance, especially with high-risk women. I felt like my doctors were much less likely to take a wait-and-see approach because of my BRCA mutation. Sure, you get to keep your breasts, but we will mash them into mammogram machines, slide you into MRI machines and stick long thick needles in your breasts or cut out a tissue samples of suspicious masses until you cry uncle, or just cry.

One of my first false alarms came after my mammogram in November 2008—the appointment where I filled out the risk assessment for hereditary breast and ovarian cancer—revealed "clustered calcifications" in my right breast. Calcifications are calcium deposits that form in women's breast tissue. They look like tiny white specks on the mammogram and are normal. When they are seen in clusters, though, that can signal a problem.

The report read, "The breast tissue is moderately dense, which may lower the sensitivity of mammography.

"There are no suspicious masses. There are clustered, heterogeneous right breast calcifications, upper outer quadrant."

Impression: Suspicious

Recommendation: Right breast stereotactic biopsy.

After identifying me as high risk, even though I hadn't taken the BRCA test yet, my doctor urged me to have the biopsy as soon as possible. My appointment was on November 24, 2008—three days before Thanksgiving. I knew that meant I'd have to wait even longer than usual for my results.

A stereotactic biopsy is a procedure also known as a needle biopsy. Needle biopsies are a less invasive procedure to remove tissue to biopsy. The needle biopsy was harder for me because I had to experience the procedure awake. Mine was at the hospital where I got my mammogram. My sister-in-law went with me. After we checked in and waited in the main lobby, a nurse led us into another, smaller waiting area, where you stay until they call you for your procedure. The chairs in the inner waiting room were more cushioned and comfortable than the ones in the front waiting area. There were copies of the usual magazines on a table in the middle of the chairs to help me catch up on news about celebrities. There was also a coffee machine and water cooler. I didn't have to wait long. The nurse then took me to a changing room. This was getting to be a familiar drill: undress from the waist up. Gown open to the front. The "gowns" were soft pink short capes that tied in the front and only went to your waist.

After I was called, the nurse led me down the hallway to a room. Inside, there was a machine attached to a cushioned table with a sheet over it. The nurse or tech helped me onto the table and asked me to lie face down. There was an opening for my breasts to go through. At some point they gave me a shot in the breast that contained a local anesthetic. I squeezed my eyes shut and grabbed the sides of the table I was lying on. They raised the table so the medical team could work underneath. They used a mammogram to guide them to the suspicious area, then drew tissue with a needle. I didn't feel a thing thanks to the anesthesia. When they finished, they wrapped my breasts in a bandage that went around my chest. I would have to wait until Monday—and worry over the holiday—to get my results.

After the needle biopsy, my right breast was sore. When I could finally take off the bandaging, I knew why. My entire breast was swollen and black and blue. It looked like someone beat the hell out of it with a baseball bat. It hurt so bad, I couldn't touch it. It hurt to look at it.

I tried not to worry about the biopsy over Thanksgiving, but how can you not freak out when you know you may get a life-altering diagnosis in a few days? Somehow, though, I just didn't think I had cancer. I don't know why. I bet a lot of people who have been diagnosed with cancer have had that feeling too though.

The next week, I got good news. It was benign.

The pathology reports sound scary even when they're giving you good news. Mine said: "Fibrocystic change with florid epithelial hyperplasia. Microcalcifications present. Fibroadenomatosis. Small fibroadenoma." The doctors recommended a mammogram in six months. I looked up fibroadenomatosis. It sounds serious. Turns out it's a benign lesion.

I thought it was over.

That's when I got the letter saying that my responses to the risk assessment indicated that I would benefit from genetic counseling, which started the process that led to my BRCA test. After we got the results and found out that I have a BRCA2 mutation, in January 2009, Dr. A ordered an MRI as a precaution. I had my first MRI that February. The scheduler asked if I was claustrophobic. I didn't think so, but I'd never had an MRI. I figured I'd be okay. On the day of the exam, I went through the usual drill. I was getting good at making doctor's appointments more convenient for myself. I had figured out what clothes and shoes were the easiest for me to change in and out of. I changed into my gown and disposable teal socks with rubber grips on the bottom. I put my clothes and purse in my locker then came back into the hallway. The nurse told me I could sit in the vinyl chair against a wall across form the changing rooms. She would come back and set up my IV so they could inject me with the "contrast," a substance that makes any potential tumors more visible during the scan.

"Would you like a warm blanket?" the nurse asked as I sat there staring off into nowhere. It can get boring in these waiting situations because you have to lock up your stuff, including your phone, and have nothing to do. It was cold in the hallway.

"Sure."

She brought a soft off-white blanket and placed it on my lap. It felt like heaven as I sat in that dimly lit hallway waiting for my IV. Sometimes a small thing like a warm blanket makes a big difference. The next stop was a room across the hall with a large, round white contraption that had a narrow tube in the center. There was a long narrow table that stuck out from the tube. There was a stool for me to step up. I had to lie face down on the table. The tech gave me earplugs and headphones.

"Would you like to listen to music?"

"Sure."

"What kind?"

"What do you have?"

I chose classical. If all I had to do was lie there, I figured it could be relaxing.

The tech gave me a ball to squeeze if there was an emergency and she needed to stop the scan. My heart started beating rapidly at the idea that I might panic. She told me I'd hear clicks and noises and that soon I would feel the contrast and it might feel warm. That there would be several parts. That I should keep still. That she'd be on the other side of the window along the wall and would ask me how I was doing periodically.

She left the room. Then, like a package of meat on a supermarket conveyer belt, I was gliding into the tube-like opening of the MRI machine. As a mother of a two-year-old, who worked full time and never got enough sleep, this was a rare opportunity to zone out. I closed my eyes. I was enjoying the peace, quiet and a rare moment when I had no responsibility other than to just lie there. A loud voice interrupted the tranquility. It was muffled like the ones you order food from at a fast-food place. Something about beginning the first set. Or something. I held a thumb up to show I was okay.

Next, I felt something warm slowly moving through my body. I felt the urge to pee. I wasn't sure I hadn't peed. Hmm. Hopefully not. I closed my eyes. The music was nice. Then came the clinking and clanking and industrial noises that turned my classical string quartet into a death metal symphony. The cacophony continued. I kept my eyes closed and lay still. I felt oddly relaxed. If they'd offered, I probably would've stayed longer.

After the MRI came more waiting. I was worried. I tried to reason that it would probably be clear since the needle biopsy had come back benign. Dr. A called when I was on my way to work. I remember sitting in my car on the top of the parking garage when he called.

"The MRI showed a 'suspicious area,'" he said. He said some other things I don't remember. My brain could not get past "suspicious area."

"What does that mean?" I asked.

My heart sank. I thought the MRI was just a precaution since I had tested for the BRCA2 mutation. My previous biopsy had come back clear.

The pathology report said: "Highly suspicious area of enhancement within the deep left breast 3–4 o'clock position. This abuts the chest wall but no definite chest wall invasion is seen. Three areas of suspicious enhancement within the right breast at nine o'clock, 11 o'clock and 12 o'clock positions as described above."

Dr. A recommended an ultrasound, a test most people know for showing them their first image of their children. I went a couple weeks after the MRI. As I lay on the exam table, the tech put a blob of gel on my breast and moved the thing, kind of like a computer mouse, over it. I thought of how exciting the procedure was when I was pregnant and got to see my son for the first time. This time, I could see the monitor, which showed some light spots on the dark background. I had no idea what they meant. My imagination ran wild. I thought of a bad comedy sketch in which a surgeon pulls something out of me as if in the delivery room . . . "It's a . . . tumor!" I studied the tech's face. She looked serious. Would I be able to tell from her face if she found something? Were they trained not to show emotion? She stopped sometimes and marked a spot. I imagined that she was trying to disguise her grave concern over what she saw.

By this time, I was having severe anxiety about all the tests and what was seeming like a real possibility of cancer. I was having some pelvic pain deep in the right side, where I imagined my ovaries were. I was getting paranoid about ovarian cancer and worried about what if a tumor was already there, multiplying . . .

I made an appointment with my gynecologist. She ordered a transvaginal ultrasound, also called TVU. I'd had one years before. You lie on a table and a technician inserts a probe into your vagina. It's awkward and uncomfortable to lie there while someone is moving a wand inside you. It ended up being a small benign cyst that was nothing to worry about.

The breast ultrasound, though, did not rule out cancer. Next, Dr. A ordered another needle biopsy. This one was scheduled for March 9. It would be guided by an MRI, rather than a mammogram as in my first needle biopsy a few months earlier. Even though the previous biopsy had come out clean, this one would take a biopsy from a different area. Dr. A was being cautious, which was comforting. After the bruising last time, I was dreading the procedure. Somehow, this time, I didn't bruise as badly.

The worst part of these cancer scares is the waiting. They don't tell you right then and there that it was all a false alarm and you're fine. It can take days. Long days spent trying to focus at work or staying in the moment while playing with your child, working or cooking dinner when your mind keeps going back to agonizing over whether you have cancer and are going to die. People you told about the biopsy check in with you. You still don't have any answers. You tell as few people as possible. You find yourself trying to calm your loved ones' fears when you're shaking inside.

Dr. A said he would call as soon as he found out, and he did. I got his call on my cell phone while taking a walking break at work to try to calm down. Dr. A had good news: the pathology came back clear.

"Thank you," I said. "Thank you so much."

I couldn't stop smiling. I was feeling an incredible sense of relief.

I was trying to get the hang of dealing these false positives. The next time, I would try not to panic because I knew that this was just part of the deal. Or I could end the cycle of screenings, false alarms, biopsies and anxiety and have surgery.

The medical appointments and bills were also stressing me out. Each time I had to go to the doctor, and since they were specialists, I had at least a $50 copay. I had deductibles and coinsurance that meant I paid 20 percent of the cost of every procedure. Surveillance was costing a small fortune. On my modest newspaper reporter's salary, I was barely keeping up with the costs. Insurance premiums kept rising, as they have for everyone. The newspaper cut our pay at one point and was planning to change to a high-deductible insurance plan. Having any kind of chronic condition can keep you falling behind financially. I knew that I was lucky to have enough to get my screenings.

The tests, appointments and biopsies can be very expensive. A study in the journal *Plastic and Reconstructive Surgery* estimated that surveillance can cost more in the long run than a prophylactic mastectomy. The study found that having a prophylactic bilateral mastectomy costs between $15,668 and $21,342, depending on the type of reconstruction involved, which is less over a lifetime than surveillance.[2] Despite this finding, it's difficult to estimate which approach will be more expensive for each individual, since the expenses will depend on a variety of unknown factors including a person's insurance plan and whether any of their screenings lead to biopsies. Based on my own experience, both approaches cost several thousands of dollars over the years and put me into debt.

As costly as surveillance or risk-reducing surgery may be, they are a bargain compared to having to go through cancer treatment. Insurance companies cover preventative mastectomies for

BRCA and other high-risk patients because it saves them money. A study in *American Health and Drug Benefits* illustrates how expensive cancer treatment can be, especially in its later stages.[3] The study reviewed claims for 8,360 women. Of them, 2,300 had Stage 0 cancers, 4,425 had Stage 1 or 2, 1,134 had Stage 3 and 501 had Stage 4. The researchers compared costs a year after diagnosis and two years after diagnosis.

The average costs allowed per patient in 24 months after diagnosis were:

- Stage 0 — $71,909
- Stage 1/2 — $97,066
- Stage 3 — $159,442
- Stage 4 — $182,655

What felt like an endless round of tests, biopsies and cancer scares was getting to me. I was slipping into a depression. I've been prone to depression as long as I can remember, and it can get worse under stress. Depression sometimes feels like going through life with one of those vests you put weights in. Everything, especially huge decisions like what to do about a BRCA mutation, feels difficult. My doctor increased the dose of my antidepressant, Pristiq. I had tried antidepressants in the past with varying success. Some of the antidepressants I had tried made me sick. One made me constantly feel like I would throw up. One made me yawn all the time. Another gave me a light buzzing sensation in my head. I hated the idea of taking an antidepressant. I didn't want to need it. But Pristiq worked. The first time I took the little pink square pill, I couldn't believe how much better I felt. Pristiq's marketing materials show a sad-looking woman hunched forward. She has a wind-up knob on her back. I always thought that looked cheesy—until I tried the medication. Was this how people born with more generous serotonin levels always felt?

After the latest false alarm, I had another appointment with the oncologist, Dr. B, in May. I wanted to do what I could to be proactive. If I wasn't ready to move ahead with surgery, she advised me to take tamoxifen, which has been shown to help reduce the risk of breast cancer. I was afraid that this drug would make me miserable. Among the side effects are hot flashes. It's not easy to motivate yourself to take a medication that could significantly lower your quality of life to prevent a cancer that may never develop in the first place. I told her that I had just changed my dose of Pristiq and that I needed time to adjust. She suggested I fill the prescription and take a couple weeks to get used to the Pristiq first.

Dr. B's office also took a blood sample. It was to measure a protein in my blood called CA125. It was not considered a reliable test because other factors could also elevate the levels, but the idea was to create a baseline. If the numbers shot up, it could signal a problem. However, the numbers could rise when there's not a problem.

Once I had adjusted to my antidepressant, my doctor urged me to start Tamoxifen. I started the pills that summer. Taking tamoxifen when you don't have breast cancer is a therapy called chemoprevention. Dr. B gave me a printout that stated that the drug could come with menopausal symptoms including hot flashes and night sweats, vaginal discomfort or bleeding. The sheet also said the drug can "increase the risk of some serious and potentially life-threatening conditions, including uterine cancer, blood clots and stroke. It can also increase the risk of getting cataracts or of needing cataract surgery."

I was scared. The hot flashes fired up within a couple of days. I felt foggy and just not right. I had pain in my pelvic area that started two weeks after I took it. My gynecologist did a pelvic exam but did not see any problem. Still, I was scared. I needed to be able to focus at work. I got a taste of what it's like to live without estrogen and it sucked. I wanted to stop taking a drug that made me miserable that I was taking to prevent a disease I didn't have. My experience on tamoxifen made me think hard about having my ovaries removed so I wouldn't need the medication anymore.

Although many doctors consider preventative mastectomies a personal decision, mine did not hesitate to tell me when I tested positive for a BRCA mutation to have my ovaries removed ASAP, since I was in my early 40s and did not plan to have more children. Research suggests that some ovarian cancers in BRCA mutation carriers may begin in the fallopian tubes, which is why they usually remove the fallopian tubes too.[4]

Some women also have hysterectomies as part of the surgery. Removing the ovaries throws you into what's called "surgical menopause," a sudden jolt to the system as it faces estrogen withdrawal. In normal menopause, women experience a gradual decline in estrogen production. Normal menopause, with its hot flashes, night sweats and mood changes, is like slowly wading into the pool. With surgical menopause, you're pushed right in. Surgical menopause can result in severe hot flashes, vaginal dryness, sexual dysfunction, sleep disturbances and cognitive changes.[5] Dr. B told me that I would not be able to take hormone therapy unless my gynecological oncologist approved it. Thankfully, he did. Research has shown that it is safe for most women with BRCA mutations to have short-term hormone therapy after risk-reducing surgery up to normal menopause age, around age 50.[6, 7]

Ovarian cancer is sometimes called a stealth cancer because many women do not notice any symptoms until it has spread throughout their bodies. Its symptoms are vague, including bloating. I get bloated every month during my period. How would anyone know whether it was ovarian cancer vs. routine bloating? There's no reliable screening for ovarian cancer. Doctors can measure a protein called CA125, which can spike if you have ovarian cancer. The problem is that it may not spike and if it does, it may not be due to cancer.

Having my ovaries removed seemed like a no-brainer given the high risk that the BRCA2 mutation brings and a family history of ovarian cancer. The more I thought about it, the more I worried that I might already have ovarian cancer. My doctor said they find it in some high-risk patients during preventative surgeries. My own health history was full of gynecological problems. I had surgery to remove painful uterine fibroids in my early 30s and painful periods and PMS that made me seriously consider a hysterectomy and bilateral salpingo-oophorectomy. Preventive oophorectomy reduced the risk of ovarian, fallopian tube and peritoneal cancer by as much as 80 percent in women with BRCA mutations, according to a 2014 study in the *Journal of Clinical Oncology*.[8] The surgery does not eliminate the risk altogether because surgeons cannot remove all the ovarian tissue in our bodies. Some of the related tissue is found in the peritoneum, a thin tissue that lines the abdomen. The risk of peritoneal cancer is low but that didn't stop me from worrying about it.[9] Removing the ovaries by age 40 also may decrease the breast cancer risk in women with BRCA mutations by as much as 50 percent, according to research.[10] (However, my doctor doubted I would get substantial breast cancer risk reduction from the surgery since I was already in my early 40s and my estrogen supply was decreasing anyway.)

I got referrals for a few different gynecological oncologists that spring.

"You need to have this surgery," Dr. D said. "Your risk is as much as 30 times higher than the average woman's."

Dr. A also urged me to have my ovaries removed. He emphasized the difficulty of catching ovarian cancer early.

"I just went to the funeral of a beautiful woman, only in her 50s, who had ovarian cancer," he said, looking grim and shaking his head.

The surgery would take one and a half hours. I'd spend two days in the hospital and need three weeks for recovery. I told my doctor that I was worried about peritoneal cancer.

"It's extremely rare," Dr. C said. He said the chances of getting it are 1–2 percent. That might be rare, but I thought of being in a room with 100 women. One or two of us would get peritoneal cancer. That was enough to fuel my anxiety. We sat in Dr. C's office. I looked down and slightly shook my head as if I just couldn't decide to go ahead and buy that new car. Why the hesitation? It wasn't a hard decision. I just didn't want to do it.

I thought maybe I could put off the surgery. Once again, I was so confused about what to do. I posted a question on the FORCE message board:

> *Ooph for BRCA2+ at age 42?*
>
> *I'm 42, BRCA2+ and had decided to go ahead with the ooph this fall. Now I'm getting scared. The info showing the risk of OC for BRCA2+ is pretty low before age 50 makes me think "why not wait?" But I'm also terrified of getting OC. It's a tough decision. Anyone have advice?*

Within five minutes, I had a response.

> *I would consider your family history. Has anyone else in your family had ovarian cancer and if so at what age? Also, would*

you be able to go on some form of hormone replacement if needed? Have you used birth control pills at least five years or more because this may lower your risk of ovarian cancer? Lots to think about. Just some ideas.

Kim, there are also specific mutations of BRCA2 that have a higher risk than the overall average BRCA2 risk, so you may want to google if yours is one of them. Sometimes I wonder if I should have waited until age 40 (had it at 45, now am 46), but knowing how I am, every backache or bloating day would be OC in my mind. So, it also depends on your nerves, so to speak.

You should check out your mutation, and family history. my doc said that at age 44, my ovaries wouldn't work that much longer anyway. the radiology ondol said it was a no brainer, given the fact the ovarian cancer is hard to spot at early stages. I had it at age 44. after I had my children. that being said, it was just another thing my then husband couldn't deal with.

BRCA2 runs in my family, both BC and OC. My doctors wanted my ovaries out at 40 because of family history and cysts. I wanted to wait until 50. I got BC at 44. If I had had my ovaries out when my doctor wanted me to, I might not have gotten BC.

After reading the responses, I realized there was no good reason to wait. Once I decided to move forward, I had to decide whether to have a hysterectomy in addition to the bilateral salpingo-oophorectomy. Different gynecological oncologists had different recommendations. In the end, I went with a surgeon who recommended a total abdominal hysterectomy and bilateral salpingo-oophorectomy. My doctor said the hysterectomy made sense for me because I had a history of painful fibroids and heavy, painful periods. He cautioned that 10–15 percent of cases have microscopic cancer, which gave me something new to worry about.

I scheduled the surgery for October 2009, less than a year after I had discovered my BRCA status. I had to take a six-week medical leave from work. Insurance would cover the surgery, though I'd have to pay my co-pays and 20 percent of the cost. I didn't have the money saved up but fortunately I could afford a payment plan. I told few people why I was having the hysterectomy/bilateral salpingo-oophorectomy. Hysterectomies are so common, nobody questions why a woman over 40 would have one.

As October 22, the day of surgery, approached, I got more and more nervous. Did I really need to do this? Could I wait? At about that time, my mom did some digging and discovered that her great-aunts had died of ovarian cancer rather than liver and stomach cancers as we previously thought.

After hearing that, I felt more confident than ever that I was doing the right thing.

I had to check in for surgery at 5:30 a.m. My mom took me. My husband stayed with our son, who was two at the time. I brought a little light blue photo album filled with pictures of Leo to keep with me at the hospital. I kept thinking of what Dr. C said, that preventative surgeries end up finding cancer in some cases. Over the past few weeks I had imagined that I was bloated, or that any gas was a sign. The waiting period before the surgery seemed to take forever. They had to ask a lot of questions. What is your full name? What medications do you take? Finally, the anesthesiologist came. My mom said I had a rough time in the recovery room and that I was crying, which is common after anesthesia. I don't remember any of it. All I remember is waking up in my hospital bed and being starving. I couldn't eat for hours. Finally, they brought food. It might have been a veggie burger; I can't remember for sure. I remember thinking the hospital food was delicious and I scarfed it down. Soon after though, I threw it up. My painkillers were making me sick. They didn't even work; I was in a lot of pain. I got queasy looking at the metal staples along my "bikini line." It was the same incision of my C-section and a surgery I had to remove a fibroid years before that caused heavy bleeding. I was having severe anxiety. I couldn't sleep. I was miserable. The nurses made me get up and walk. I spent three nights in the hospital. My husband brought our son, but I couldn't hold him or let him near my pelvic area.

Dr. C wanted me to try not taking any hormones. I was scared. I'd read horror stories about surgical menopause on the message boards. I experienced hot flashes on Tamoxifen. I could only imagine how terrible surgical menopause felt for some women. I wanted to try going hormone-free though. Doctors prescribe Effexor, an antidepressant, to women for menopause symptoms. Since I was already taking Pristiq, I thought maybe my medication would offset any problems.

Wrong.

Within a couple days after I got home from the hospital, I was having severe hot flashes. I'd wake up in a pool of sweat. It's jarring to wake up in a cold, wet bed. Other times, I'd be freezing and pull a comforter over me. This won't last forever, I thought. This will pass. I tried to calm myself. Over the next couple of days, I felt worse. In addition to the hot flashes and night sweats, I felt foggy, out of it and unable to focus. I was on medical leave, so all I had to do was rest, but I couldn't even read. After being home for about a week, I went to the doctor for a post-surgery visit.

"How are you doing?" the nurse asked.

"I don't feel well," I said, explaining the symptoms.

The nurse said it takes time to get used to the lack of estrogen. I could not imagine how this could get better. I had no energy. It felt like the life force had been sucked out of me.

Dr. C examined me and said everything was healing well. Thankfully the pathology showed there was no cancer. He left the room. The nurse told me I could change back into my clothes. I went into the little changing room in the examination room and got dressed. I went into the hall to check out. I stood at the counter as the woman at the desk looked up my account. I gripped the counter. I felt like I was going to faint.

"I think I need to sit down," I said.

The nurse led me back to the exam room. I lay down on the exam table for several minutes. I was sweating and breathing as if I'd just climbed four flights of stairs. Dr. C came in and wrote me a prescription for a low dose of estradiol. I lay there for a few more minutes.

My husband and son had been killing time in the office building while I was at my appointment. When they came to pick me up, I heard the nurse bring them down the hallway to the exam room I was in. They helped me get up from the exam table and we left. We filled the prescription on the way home. Within hours of taking one of the pills, I felt like I was coming back to life. The difference was dramatic. Dr. C said I could take my estradiol until about normal menopause age. So, I had a few years to go. By the next week's post-op appointment, I was feeling human again. Once my hormones were under control, I recovered over the next several weeks and got back to regular life. As far as a double mastectomy, I wasn't close to being ready.

By the end of 2009, I had recovered from my surgery and was back to my normal routine. After the ordeal of having my ovaries removed, I needed time before considering another surgery.

Over the next couple of years, I had other problems to deal with. My marriage was not working out. My BRCA situation had little to do with it other than adding to a huge pile of stressors that included financial setbacks, adjusting to being new parents, dealing with various health issues and working in an industry that seemed to be in a death spiral. I fell into a depression. We went to counseling and ended up divorcing in 2012. Leo was five. We kept things amicable and focused on doing what was best for him. As if divorce and health issues were not enough, I also was grieving what felt like the slow death of my journalism career. I had discovered journalism in college and fell in love with being able to apply my love of writing to news and issues that mattered. After 21 years as a newspaper reporter, my career looked bleaker than ever as round after round of layoffs hit *The Dallas Morning News*. The newspaper industry continued to implode as newspaper circulation and advertising revenue steadily fell year after year. *The News* had cut my pay and benefits and many good journalists and friends had lost their jobs. That fall, another round of layoffs loomed over us. Even if I survived this blow, I felt like another round would get me like the monster that keeps coming back in a horror movie. The idea of retiring in the industry seemed farfetched. Too many colleagues had been laid off in their 50s and 60s before they were ready to retire and after it was difficult to start in a new direction and I decided to jump ship. I mentioned to a couple of acquaintances that I may be looking for a job, which led to an offer to work as communications director for a nonprofit that helps people experiencing homelessness. I decided to leave journalism and try a new direction.

BRCA went on the backburner. Other than getting my regular screenings, I didn't obsess over it, maybe because there was only so much I could deal with at a time. Thankfully, I did not have any more cancer scares. Dr. A said the initial MRIs and mammograms would set a baseline that radiologists could use to compare the results of future screenings. He predicted that I would face fewer false alarms because the previous screenings would help radiologists better identify problem areas versus false alarms. I didn't visit FORCE's message boards or think too much about BRCA as I struggled to deal with divorce and a career change. Fear of cancer was always there, though, in the back of my mind. I felt like I was buying time or getting away with something that would not last. I didn't want to have to worry about more false alarms, biopsies and anxiety. I was leaning toward having The Surgery. Probably. Someday.

PATIENT COPY
Comprehensive BRACAnalysis®
BRCA1 and BRCA2 Analysis Result

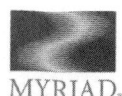

MYRIAD.

PHYSICIAN	SPECIMEN		PATIENT	
	Specimen Type:	**Blood**	Name:	**Horner, Kimberly**
	Draw Date:	**Jan 07, 2009**	Date of Birth:	
	Accession Date:	**Jan 08, 2009**	Patient ID:	
	Report Date:	**Jan 12, 2009**	Gender:	**Female**
			Accession #:	**00443844-BLD**
			Requisition #:	**1293847**

Test Results and Interpretation

POSITIVE FOR A DELETERIOUS MUTATION

Test Performed	Result	Interpretation
BRCA1 sequencing	No Mutation Detected	No Mutation Detected
5-site rearrangement panel	No Mutation Detected	No Mutation Detected
BRCA2 sequencing	8803delC	**Deleterious**

Analysis consists of sequencing of all translated exons and immediately adjacent intronic regions of the BRCA1 and BRCA2 genes and a test for five specific BRCA1 rearrangements.

The results of this analysis are consistent with the germline BRCA2 mutation 8803delC, resulting in premature truncation of the BRCA2 protein at amino acid position 2862. Although the exact risk of breast and ovarian cancer conferred by this specific mutation has not been determined, studies of this type of mutation in high-risk families indicate that deleterious mutations in BRCA2 may confer as much as an 84% risk of breast cancer and a 27% risk of ovarian cancer by age 70 in women (Am. J. Hum. Genet. 62:676-689, 1998). Mutations in BRCA2 have been reported to confer a 12% risk of a second breast cancer within five years of the first (J Clin Oncol 17:3396-3402, 1998), as well as a 16% risk of subsequent ovarian cancer (J Natl Cancer Inst 91:1310-1315, 1999). This mutation may also confer up to a 6% risk of male breast cancer by age 70 and 20% risk of prostate cancer by age 80 (J Natl Cancer Inst 91:1310-1315, 1999), as well as increased (albeit low) risks of some other cancers. Each first degree relative of this individual has a one-in-two chance of having this mutation. Family members can be tested for this specific mutation with a single site analysis.

Please contact Myriad Professional Support at 1-800-469-7423 to discuss any questions regarding this result.

Test result from Myriad Genetics diagnosing my BRCA2 mutation.

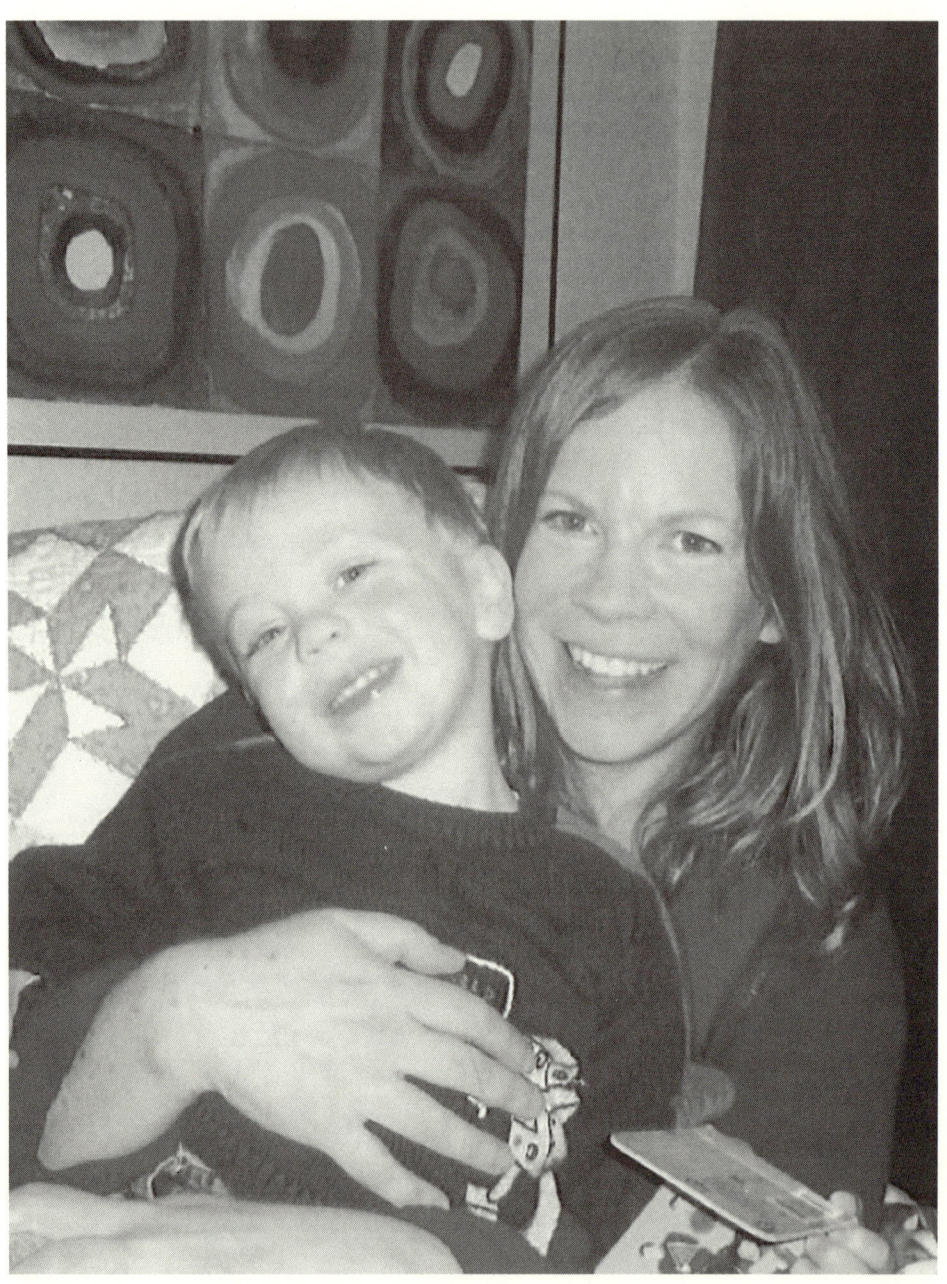

Me with Leo, my son (age 1), in 2009, the year I found out I carried a BRCA2 mutation that drastically increased my risk of breast and ovarian cancers.

A family history filled with cancer

My family tree on my mother's side includes multiple cases of breast, ovarian and pancreatic cancers, shown here by type of cancer and age of death.

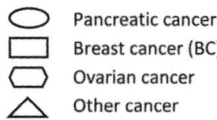

Pancreatic cancer
Breast cancer (BC)
Ovarian cancer
Other cancer

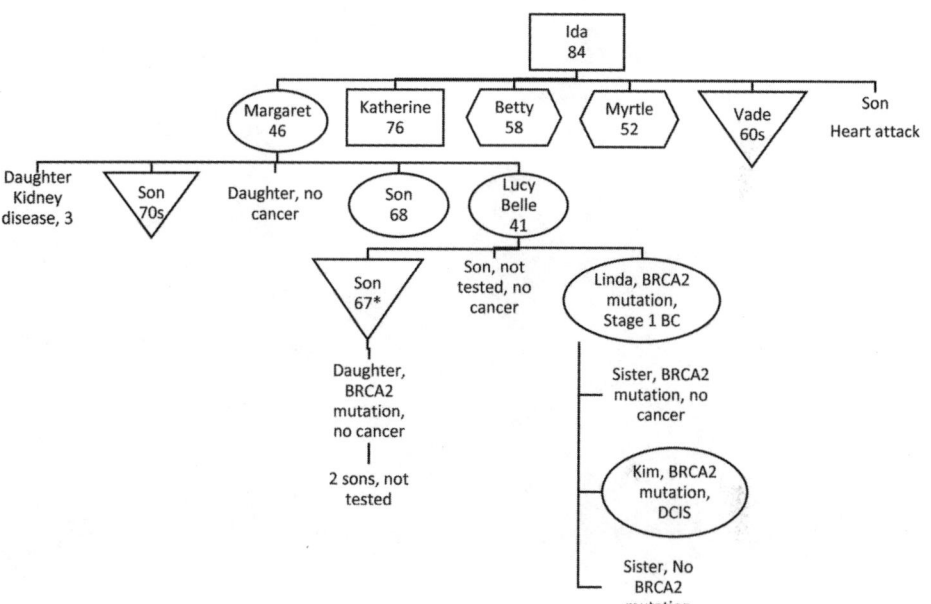

*BRCA2 mutation, bladder cancer, died of other causes.

Family History chart

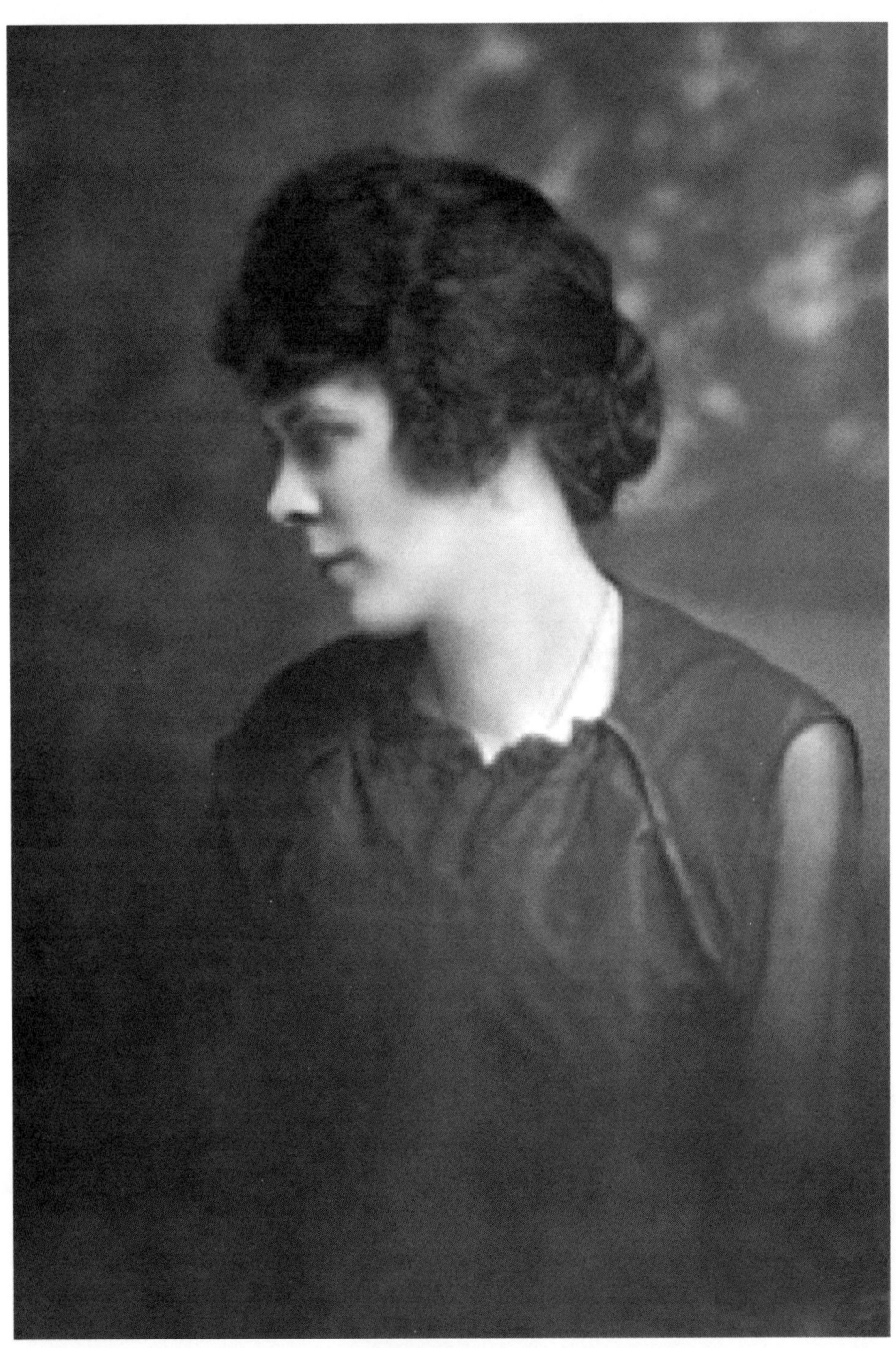

Margaret, my great-grandmother, who died of breast cancer when she was 46.

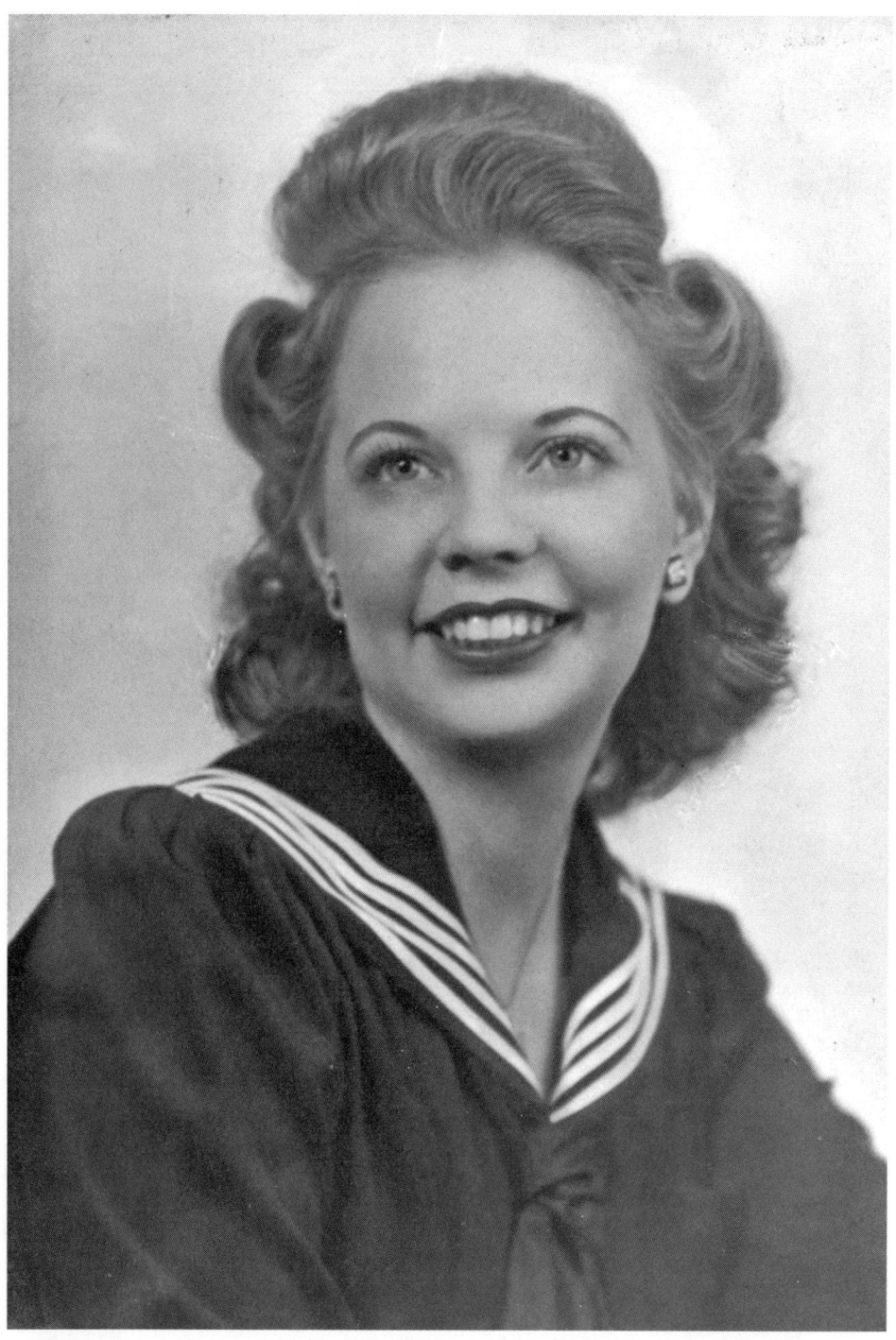

Lucy, my grandmother, died of breast cancer when she was only 41, leaving three devastated children.

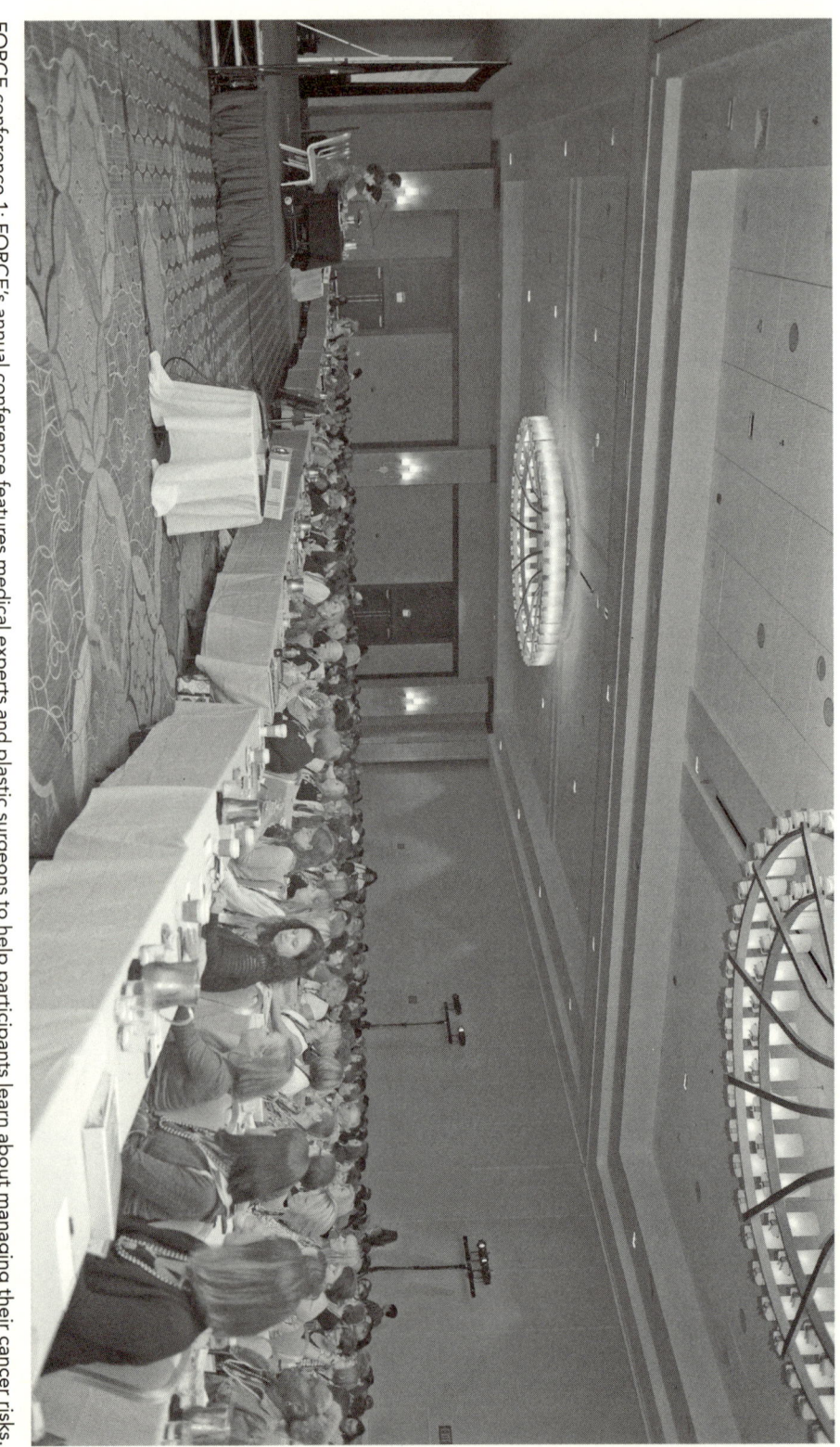

FORCE conference 1: FORCE's annual conference features medical experts and plastic surgeons to help participants learn about managing their cancer risks. Courtesy of FORCE.

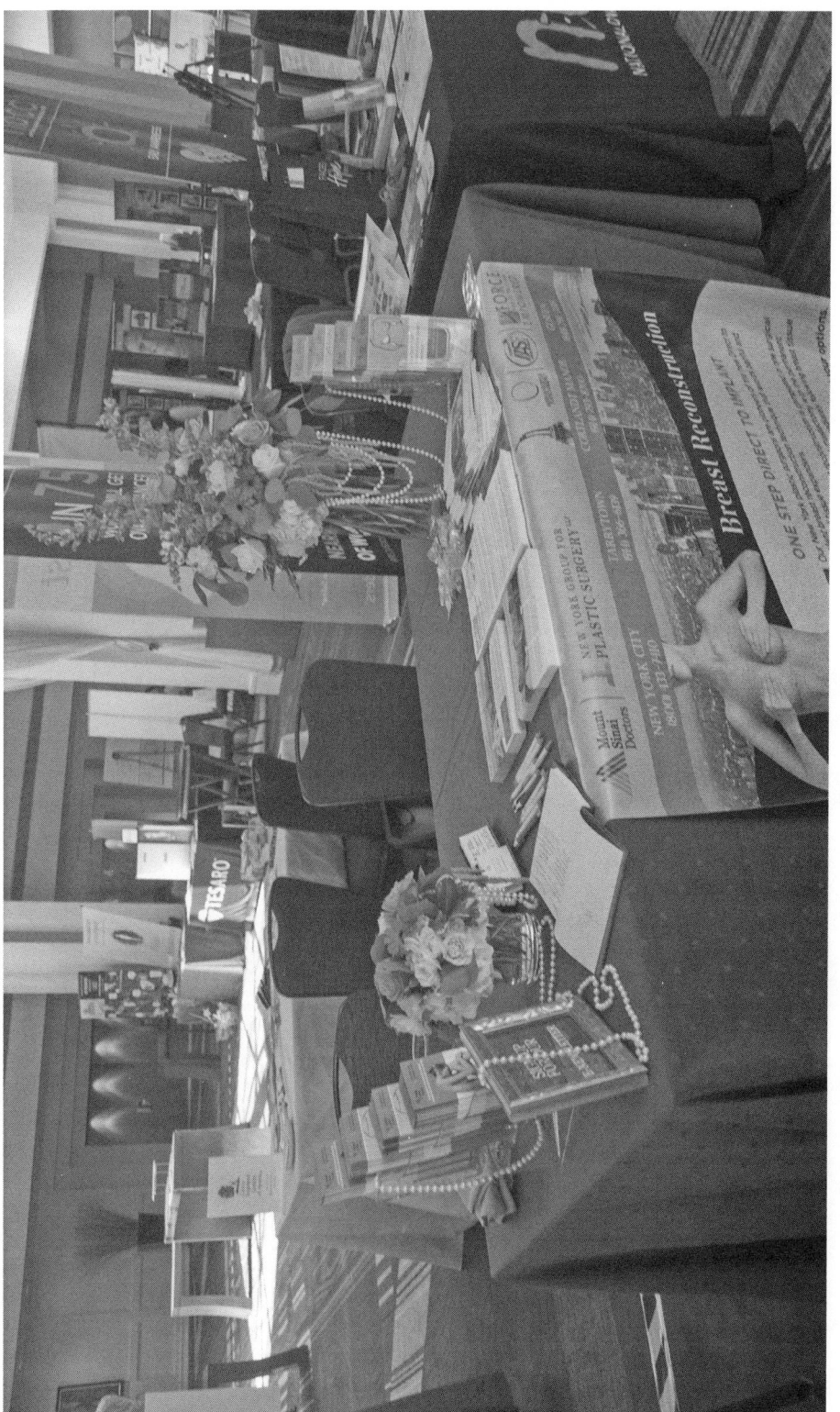

FORCE conference 2: Exhibitor's hall at the FORCE conference. Courtesy of FORCE

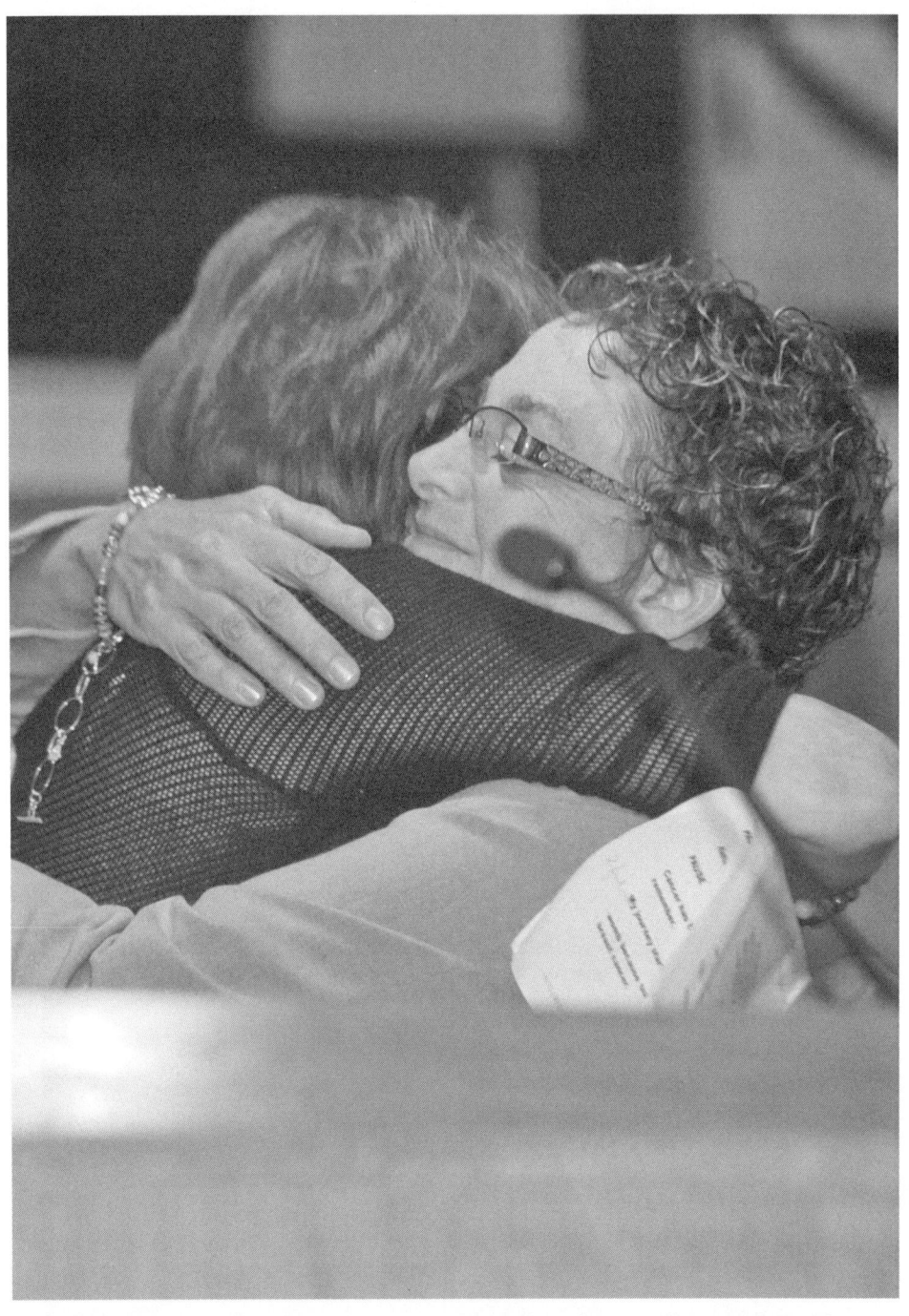

FORCE—Sue Friedman hugs participant at annual FORCE conference. *Courtesy of FORCE*

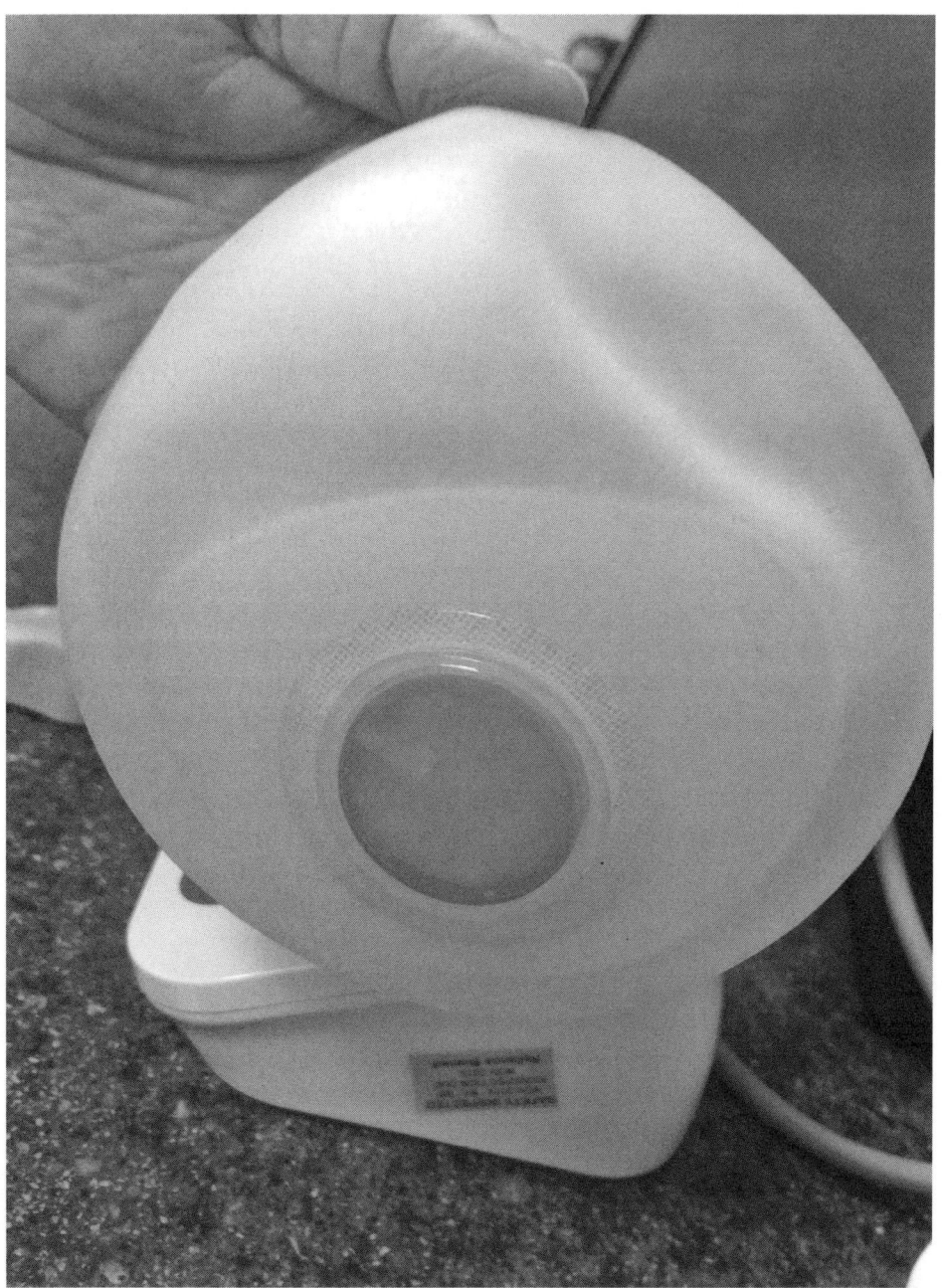

Expander (photo taken at my doctor's office). This is what an expander looks like. After my mastectomies, my plastic surgeon put these in my chest and then, over several visits between June and September, filled the device with a small amount of saline to slowly expand my skin before exchanging them for the implants.

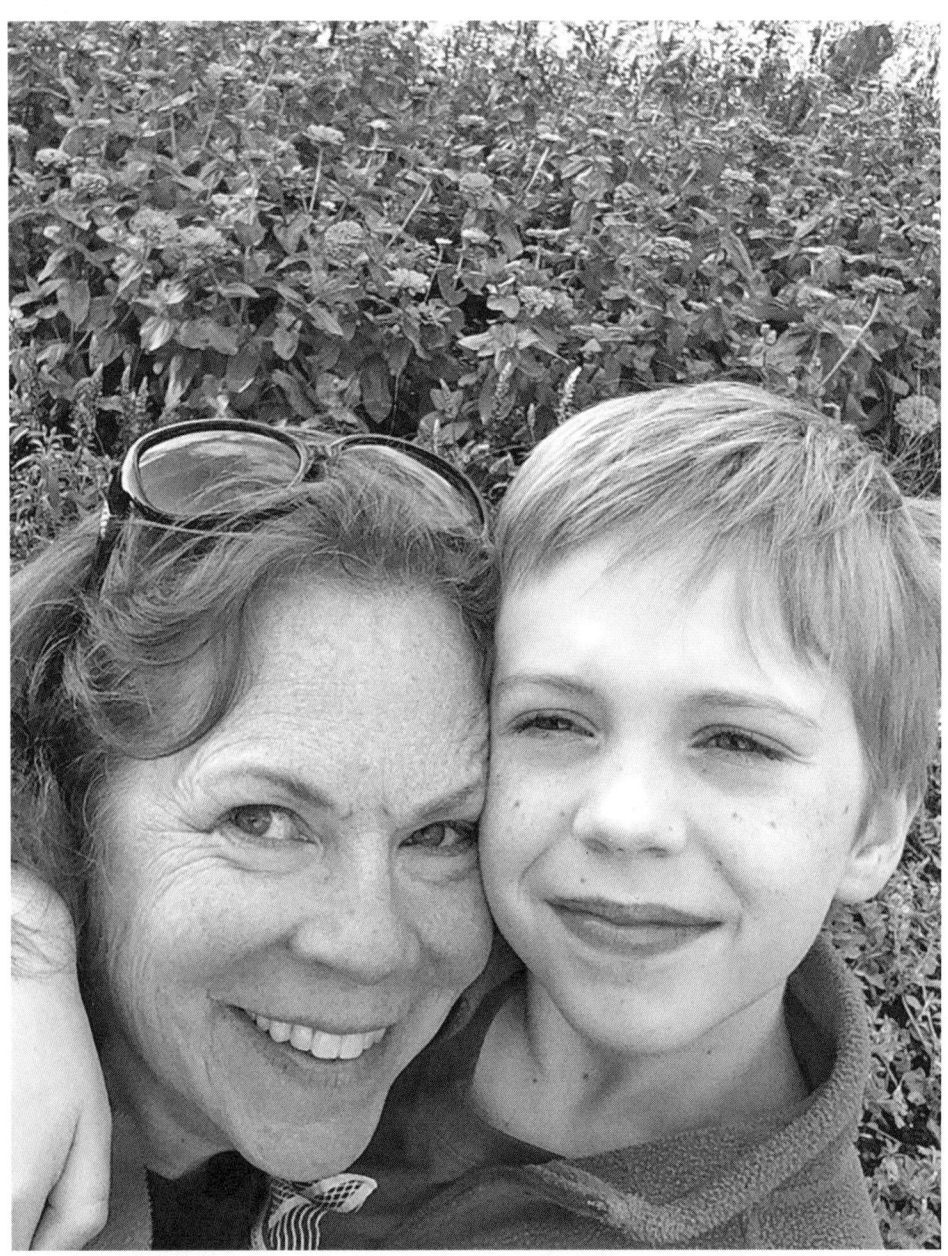

Kim and her son, Leo, in 2016, after she recovered from a bilateral mastectomy.

CHAPTER 6

The Push

"Having breast cancer is massive amounts of no fun. First, they mutilate you; then they poison you; then they burn you. I have been on blind dates better than that."[1]

—Molly Ivins, diagnosed with Stage 3 breast cancer in 1999, died in 2007

I had pretty much decided that I should have The Surgery. But it would take a push.

That came in 2015, when my mom was diagnosed with breast cancer. Until then, she had defied genetics. After watching her mom die of breast cancer and two great-aunts die of other cancers when she was growing up, my mom was diligent about getting screenings.

Her first breast cancer scare had come in 1984 when she was 39—about the same age her mother was diagnosed with breast cancer. Her physician's assistant had thought she felt a mass on the right breast and brought in the doctor to look. The doctor felt a mass too. They referred her to get a mammogram, which was a relatively new procedure at that time. She had never had one before. The results were inconclusive. Her doctor terrified my mom by telling her he thought it was malignant. Thankfully, mom got a second opinion. That doctor said the lump felt more like a cyst. And thankfully, a biopsy showed that was all it was.

She had another scare in 2014, when a mammogram detected a suspicious spot. The sonogram could not determine whether it was a mass, so she had a needle biopsy, which turned out benign. Given the good results, she was not concerned when she went in for a mammogram the next year, in 2015. She had not felt any lumps. Neither had her doctor on a routine clinical breast exam. However, the mammogram indicated another suspicious area. The tech who performed the test was diligent in getting a full picture of the area near the breast bone, since that was the area that had been biopsied the previous year. Mom had to have another biopsy.

This time, it was cancer.

The tumor was 1.5 cm.—smaller than a dime. Fortunately, it had not spread to her lymph nodes. She was diagnosed with Stage 1 breast cancer. The tumor was ER-positive, which means it had estrogen receptors. The type of breast cancer helps doctors determine the best treatment. She had to choose between a lumpectomy and mastectomy. She and her doctor decided a lumpectomy, a simpler surgery, was the best option at the time. My mom has other health issues and the concern was that less surgery was best. Since it was a small tumor, my mom's breast surgeon told her she did not think she would need chemotherapy. This was good news because we worried that chemo would be especially difficult for her given her health. The lumpectomy went well. The surgeon removed one lymph node, which tested negative for cancer.

Then we got some bad news. The pathology showed that mom's tumor was a fast-growing type. Her oncologist was recommending chemo. Mom was terrified. Her doctor convinced her she would handle it okay. They installed a port in her chest area on a Monday. She started treatment the next day. Mom felt fine the first two days. It seemed like chemo might be manageable. By that Thursday, though, she felt miserable. Her stomach was bloated, she couldn't sleep, and she was in extreme pain on her left side. She ended up in the ER on that Saturday. Doctors diagnosed her with severe diverticulitis. She spent five days in the hospital. Every time I visited, she was in pain and in tears. Later, she said she thought she was going to die. She vowed no more chemo.

Her oncologist told her she was making a mistake. He painted a doom-and-gloom scenario.

"He said I most likely had cancer in my body," she said. "He said, 'You could still have cancer come back.'" She got a second opinion. It couldn't have been more different from the first one. The next oncologist told her she was "cancer free."

Mom's hair started falling out soon after the chemo. Her white hair had been short but full and a little spiky. Now hardly any was left. The hair loss may be the least physically painful chemo side effect, but one of the most visible signs of what's going on inside. Luckily, there are seemingly infinite options to cover your head. Mom bought a cute pink close-fitting cap. Then she decided to get a wig.

The wig shop was in a strip mall next to a diner. Inside, you could see rows and rows of mannequin heads with thick, full hair from short to long, curly to straight and brunette to blonde. In the middle of the small store, there were places to sit in front of a mirror to try them on. The staff counseled us on what would and would not be covered by insurance. The wigs weren't cheap. Even the ones with synthetic hair cost at least $400 just for a decent-looking one. Mom chose a sandy blonde wig with a stylish short layered cut that always looked like she had just stepped out of a salon. She wore the wig all the time and looked great. She got tons of compliments on it. Only downside was it felt hot. Underneath, she was bald until her hair slowly grew back in from short stubbles to her previous short hairstyle.

That fall, mom switched doctors again. Her new oncologist recommended she get a double mastectomy because the BRCA2 mutation put her at a high risk of getting another breast cancer. We had several mother-daughter outings to consultations with breast surgeons and plastic surgeons, followed by visits to our favorite pancake spot to at least get something fun out of the trip. After what mom had been through, I was starting to seriously consider having a preventative double mastectomy sooner than later.

When we met with Dr. E in the fall of 2015. I knew I wanted to go with him. So did mom. We had heard him speak at a Genetic Counselors' Conference in Dallas and liked him a lot. Dr. E has a bright personality. He's so energetic; he sort of bounces in the room. He's so upbeat and friendly, it almost doesn't feel like you're talking about having your breast tissue removed and a fake substitute put in. He explained that after the breast surgeon removes my breast tissue, he'd put in what's called an expander. The expander helps slowly stretch your skin to make room for the implants. Dr. E would fill it a small amount at a time over a period of months until it reaches the size of breasts I want. Then, he would do an "exchange" surgery, which means replacing the expanders with the permanent breast implants. I tried to calm myself by thinking the surgeons just make a small opening, scoop out some tissue, and put in an expander. No big deal, right?

"What size do you want to go with? You could do a C cup," he said.

"I keep telling her to go big," my mom said, trying to get me to laugh.

"I think I want to stay about the same," I said. "Maybe just a little bit bigger."

Dr. E said I could do a deep inferior epigastric perforator, or DIEP flap, a surgery that would transfer fat, skin and blood vessels from the wall of my lower belly and move them to rebuild my chest. Of course, you need extra fat tissue in your stomach to do that. I looked down at my gut. Much to my frustration, I was struggling with stomach fat. In the past few years, fat seemed to accumulate there more than ever. I exercised and (mostly) ate well, but the damn thing wasn't going away. I told Dr. E I was concerned about a DIEP. I had seen the scars involved. They go from one side of your waist to the other. I'd seen a photo at a conference and it was painful just to think about it.

Dr. E looked at my stomach.

"Stand up," he said. He studied my stomach for a moment, then declared what no woman should ever have to hear.

"You have enough stomach tissue to form two small breasts," he said.

I saw my face squish up in the mirror. I was teetering in that place where I could burst into either tears or laughter. At least he didn't say I had enough stomach fat to form huge breasts.

I had a bunch of questions.

Could I get a "one-step" surgery? It was a big thing on the FORCE boards. Some doctors will put in the implant immediately after the breast surgeon does the mastectomy instead of expanders. *No. It's possible in some cases but usually it doesn't get a good result and needs revisions.*

Do you recommend saline or silicone? *Silicone.* Are silicone implants safe? *Yes.* How long does the surgery take? *About six hours.* How long would the expander process take? *Three-to four months, possibly longer.* How long would I need to take off work? *Three weeks.* How far before the surgery would I need to schedule? *A couple months.*

What kind of follow-up or screening would I need after the surgery? *Your breast surgeon would do clinical exams.* I wouldn't need mammograms ever again. Okay, that's a huge plus to never have to get your breasts literally squished between two large plates while you worry about how much tighter the technician could possibly turn the knob that squeezes the plates together.

You could still get breast cancer after a risk-reducing mastectomy, but the odds are low. Doctors say any lump would be felt on the surface. There would not be any danger of cancer underneath the implant because the breast tissue is gone.

Several studies have noted that women who got breast cancer after a risk-reducing mastectomy had a specific type of mastectomy that left behind breast tissue. "Almost all new breast cancers after bilateral prophylactic mastectomy occur in patients who had significant breast tissue remaining, such as those who underwent subcutaneous mastectomy and those who had residual tissue in the axillary tail after surgery," according to a 2017 article in the *Annals of Surgical Oncology*.[2]

I had a hard time imagining myself with breast implants. Until that point, I would've never believed you if you told me I would be considering them. I'd always associated implants with abnormally large and abnormally perky round stripper or *Baywatch* breasts. I didn't understand why anyone would want them—or the type of man who would like you better if you had bigger boobs. I thought it was sad that anyone would have a couple of blobs of silicone surgically implanted so they could conform to some stupid standard of beauty. And now here I was, considering having blobs of silicone surgically implanted in my body. Part of me thought I should just go flat—no implants. Why put anything in there at all? The fake boobs would be purely cosmetic. Would it be braver to just say no? Maybe a more evolved person wouldn't care. I did though. I knew I would feel self-conscious about not having boobs. I thought that reconstruction would help me look and feel more "normal," whatever that is, because I was feeling anything but. One day, I hope there will be options that will make it seem archaic and ridiculous that women ever had blobs of plastic-covered gel implanted in their chests. For now, well, foobs just seemed like the best option.

After Dr. E left, the nurse came in. She showed us an expander. It's a round plastic blob that feels squishy like one of those soft, silicone containers for salad dressing. It's bigger and more the size and shape of a hamburger bun. There's a plastic piece on it with a mechanism to allow the staff to insert a needle and fill it with saline.

They keep things moving in surgery offices. Next, a woman holding a professional camera knocked lightly and came into the room. It was time for my photo shoot. I wasn't expecting this. They led me to a room down the hall, a photo studio of sorts. There were several markings on the floor at different angles. The photographer asked me to stand on a marked spot in the middle. I was wearing my black pants and shoes. From the waist up, it was just the white gown I'd become so familiar with. She asked me to take it off. By this time, I had been to so many doctors and had to show them my chest so many times, I was starting to become less self-conscious.

She took some photos of me facing straight ahead. Then turn slightly right, turn again, then to the left. The camera clicked. I imagined myself trying a sexy model pout for the camera. The photographer directed me to stand on another one of the masking tape markings. I was getting used to having my breasts inspected as if they were no different a body part than an ear or foot, but this was new for me. It was the first time I'd ever posed for topless photos.

"We're done," she said after a dozen shots. She picked a clipboard from a counter and handed it to me.

"Would you be willing to sign a form giving permission for your photos to be used in research?" the nurse asked. She said the photos do not show my face, only my breasts.

"Sure," I said. Why not. It was weird to think about medical students looking at photos of my breasts. By now, who knows how many medical students have seen them.

One of the big decisions involved in reconstruction is whether to keep your nipples. That's what they call a nipple-sparing mastectomy. It's something you never imagine yourself contemplating. It's not an option for everyone; it depends on different factors including your anatomy. My plastic surgeon said I was a candidate for the procedure.

I asked the breast surgeon if it was safe. If not, I didn't want nipples that bad. Studies increasingly have shown that keeping your nipples does not raise your risk of cancer.[3] My breast surgeon said removing my nipples would not make a significant difference in my risk. So I decided that if I was going to lose my breasts, I would at least hang on to my nipples.

After going through with consultations with breast surgeons and plastic surgeons, having my photos taken and talking about specifics about the surgery, I was getting freaked out about the possibility that I might do this thing. My mind raced to find anything and everything possible to worry about. A 2014 study about complications after nipple-sparing mastectomy found that 12 percent of patients faced scary-sounding complications such as nipple necrosis.[4]

I'd read on the FORCE message boards about skin rippling over implants, infections and other issues people faced. From what I had read, it seemed reasonable to expect some revisions or at least mild complications. Reading message boards can make the likelihood of complications seem worse than the reality, however, because they often draw people who are having the most problems and need support.

Of all the things to worry about, complications were lower down the list. I was much more afraid of The Surgery itself. I chose my surgeons and decided on nipple-sparing reconstruction with implants. The only thing left was to set a date.

Mom planned her surgery quickly. She had a double mastectomy in November 2015. She planned to have implants then decided not to go through with reconstruction on the morning of the surgery. She did not want to risk any more pain and complications than necessary. Mom's pathology came back with a surprise: she had breast cancer in her other breast. The tumor did not show up on a recent mammogram. It was .08 cm. It had not spread to her lymph nodes. Mom did not need any further treatment after the mastectomy. Now, all she has to do is see the breast surgeon and oncologist for checkups every six months. The fact that screening had missed her other breast cancer and her experience with Stage 1 cancer and chemotherapy reinforced my concerns about screenings and about the implications of even an early-stage cancer. Once you've had cancer, there's the fear that it will come back or that it never completely went away. Even after treatment, no one can promise the cancer won't return or spread to another part of the body. Whenever she has an ache or pain, she thinks of the doom-and-gloom scenario one of her oncologists painted and worries that her cancer could have spread to her bones. Thankfully, that has not happened. To me, the risk of recurrence after a cancer diagnosis, even an early stage one, was another selling point for having mastectomies *before* a cancer diagnosis.

At the same time, another woman in our family, my sister's mother-in-law, Sally, was dying of breast cancer. She had been diagnosed with early stage breast cancer more than a decade earlier. At that time, she had a double mastectomy with reconstruction using tissue from her abdomen. She had chemotherapy and took tamoxifen for five years. After that, she was fine for several years. She was a petite woman who stayed active volunteering at a food pantry and playing golf, traveling and enjoying her grandsons. She had her annual mammogram each January and her last one had been clean. She had aches and pains that she associated with age. Then Sally started experiencing severe back pain. Doctors discovered a large tumor pressing against her spine; breast cancer had spread throughout her body. She spent her final weeks in the hospital in immense pain. She died in December 2015, less than a year after her symptoms began. She was 75.

I'd seen too much suffering from breast cancer. I decided I should have The Surgery sooner rather than later.

CHAPTER 7

Just Do It

"You gain strength, courage and confidence by every experience in which you really stop to look fear in the face. You are able to say to yourself, 'I have lived through this horror. I can take the next thing that comes along.' You must do the thing you think you cannot do."[1]

—Eleanor Roosevelt

I thought a lot about scheduling The Surgery. And I thought a lot about excuses to hold off. There was this or that project at work or the class I was taking that semester. I just couldn't seem to pull the trigger. I Googled advice on how to move forward when you know what to do but feel stuck. There's no secret formula. Nike's "Just Do It" slogan says it best, but it's easier said than done. I decided to talk to a therapist. I had seen one, named Helen, during and after my divorce and made an appointment to talk to her about The Surgery. I still had a hard time talking about having a BRCA2 mutation and the idea of having a double mastectomy to anyone outside my family and others with the mutation.

One afternoon, I sat on the gray couch in Helen's office. There was a box of tissues on a stool next to me and a bookshelf with titles about depression, anxiety and other disorders. Aside from the occasional ding of the elevator down the hall, it was quiet. Helen sat in a chair across from me. I told her about the BRCA2 mutation, my high risk of breast cancer and that I've decided I need this surgery but I'm afraid and feel stuck.

"What are you afraid of?" she asked.

I paused before answering. How much time did she have?

"Everything," I said. I told her I was afraid of something going wrong with the surgery, although my surgeons are great, and it should be fine. I was afraid that I'd be in a lot of pain after and that it would be a difficult recovery. I was afraid of losing my breasts. I was afraid of how people would react. I was nervous about having to ask for so much time off at work. I didn't know what to tell people. I was nervous about how the guy I had started dating would react. A major surgery and change could feel like a lot for someone you only recently met to take on. Would I have to deal with a breakup in addition to the surgery? These fears streamed through in my head like binge watching the same annoying show over and over. They were driving me nuts.

My therapist had me take on my fears, one by one.

I said I was afraid of pain.

"But you've had surgeries before, right? And you got through them."

"Yes."

I said I was afraid of complications.

"How likely are complications?"

"They're somewhat likely, but overall I know I'm in good hands and that nothing major will go wrong with the surgery."

I said I was afraid of the awkwardness of explaining my surgery and people's reactions.

"You don't have to tell anyone why you're having surgery do you?"

"No."

I said I was afraid that the guy I was seeing could be scared off by the surgery or that it could be too much to deal with since we hadn't been seeing each other for very long.

"His response will give you some good information," she said.

As we broke down my fears, I could see that none of them was insurmountable. I may not like the outcomes, but I would survive.

During one session I got so frustrated with all the back and forth going on in my head and said: "I wish I could just cut through all this noise and do what I think is best."

"And what would that be?" Helen asked.

It only took me a second to answer: "To have the surgery."

Blurting that out felt good. It felt like a huge weight had lifted. There it was. I said it. Deep down, I knew what I needed to do. What was stopping me?

All I wanted was to do what would give me the best chance of living a long happy healthy life and watching Leo, who was eight at the time, grow up. My worst nightmare was to become terminally ill and regret that I had not done everything I could to prevent the cancer. Reducing my risk of breast cancer as much as possible made all the sense in the world through that lens. There was no other choice. Tears rolled down my face.

"I think it's beautiful that you want to do this for your son and yourself," she said.

I muttered a "thanks" between sobs.

When I thought of scheduling the surgery, I felt a wave of panic.

Helen pointed out something I hadn't considered.

"I think a lot of this is your anxiety," she said.

I knew that I had anxiety over the surgery. Who wouldn't? I hadn't considered how much, though, the anxiety itself was holding me back.

"Anxiety makes you overestimate the danger and underestimate your ability to cope with it," Helen said. "Anxiety makes us want to avoid."

Anxiety can fool you into thinking you are making a rational decision when you're just trying to avoid something.

"So how do I keep it from taking over?" I asked.

Helen suggested trying to recognize when anxiety reared its ugly head.

"It helps if you can say, 'Okay, that's just my anxiety acting up,'" she said. "Remember why you're doing this."

I wrote in my notebook to try to remember that next time. The problem is that anxiety takes over before you even realize what's happening. Anxiety can come up with a dozen reasons for not scheduling surgery and they can sound so convincing, you don't have to face the fact that you're just too afraid. I was angry at myself for being so scared and for letting my fear keep me stuck.

"It's understandable," Helen said. "I'd be concerned if you weren't worried about the surgery."

Around that time, I was dealing with a loss of estrogen. My gynecological oncologist had cut me off. I was only allowed to take it until normal menopause age. My time was up. I wondered if the lack of estrogen could be making my anxiety even worse.

I kept delaying for weeks. During one session, Helen asked: "What do you think you'll do?"

I sat on the couch, staring at the floor. I wanted to say I'd schedule the surgery. On the other hand, I didn't want to make any promises I couldn't keep. I came up with what I thought would be a good way to put things off.

"I need to think about when it would be a good time to have the surgery," I said. Would it be best when my son was in school or out on summer vacation? I was taking a class that semester. Should I wait till it was over?

Helen wasn't going to let me leave it at that.

"When would be a reasonable time to make a decision by?"

I thought, "did we have to go there?" Apparently so. I looked at my calendar.

"I don't know . . . maybe by the end of the month?"

"That sounds reasonable. Do you want to plan that?"

"Yes." I was winging it. I wrote the date down in my notebook. Ugh. I wanted to decide by then. It freaked me out though.

The end of the month came. I had another appointment with Helen coming up. I still hadn't decided. I didn't want to go to my appointment without an answer. After some thinking, I decided to try to schedule the surgery in May, when my class would be over, and things would slow down at work. The next step would be to schedule the damn thing. I was taking baby steps. Just deciding on a target date was a big step. I was feeling pretty proud of myself. I shared the big accomplishment at my next appointment with Helen.

"That's great," she said. "When will you schedule the surgery?"

I was afraid she would ask that. I told her I'd schedule it by the time I came to my next appointment in two weeks. The day of the appointment, though, I still hadn't done it. I didn't want to show up without having a date scheduled and I knew that there was no way to feel "ready" for what I was about to do. You just do it. So that morning, I forced myself to call the scheduler in the plastic surgeon's office. My heart was racing, and I felt shaky. The scheduler was business-like and anyone listening might have thought I was scheduling something as routine as a teeth cleaning. She suggested Friday, May 20, 2016. I'd have the surgery around 7:00 a.m.

And that was it.

My heart was pounding. I realized that, as usual, the dread leading up to an anxiety-provoking event is worse than the actual event. Once I had scheduled the surgery, I told my family, a few friends and my boss. I had left the nonprofit by this point and worked in the communications department at a great university. I wouldn't have minded talking about it, but somehow, I couldn't tell my coworkers about the type of surgery I was having. I knew I would start bawling if I mentioned it. Also, having a double mastectomy for preventative reasons is a weird thing to have to talk about. BRCA mutations and their risks are not well known or understood, so telling anyone about the surgery requires a little extra explanation that feels like Too Much Information. I had no idea how much to divulge and as usual, looked for guidance from others on the FORCE message board. Others had posed that question. The answers made me feel less alone in my confusion over how to handle the situation:

> *Guest: I have found that people do not understand the magnitude of the risk, nor do they even consider having to worry about breast cancer before 50, let alone before 40. They tend to think that chemo is simple, and foolproof, if they do not have close personal experience with cancer survivors.*

> *Guest: I've struggled with my role in educating people about BRCA/being a BRCA ambassador. Some days I am strong enough to take the time and other days, I am not.*

> *Guest: When I had my PBM, I let most co-workers assume I had BC (breast cancer) even though it was preventative. I was emotionally and physically too exhausted to do otherwise and it felt too personal (more personal than my relationship with them was.)*

My emotions about the surgery were exhausting. I felt lucky to have this option and to have the insurance necessary to make it within my reach (although surgery bills would take years to repay). I was also sad that I had to take such a step to try to protect my health. It was a lot to give up. I'd probably lose all sensation in my breasts. No hugs, no contact would ever be quite the same ever again. Going through the surgery and recovery would be hard. I couldn't help being scared. I stumbled upon a book that helped me see that I might feel better if I could stop the internal debate and just accept that I will have conflicting feelings. In her book, *When Things Fall Apart*, author Pema Chödrön, a Buddhist nun, writes about the need to "dissolve the dualistic struggle, our habitual tendency to struggle against what's happening to us or in us." She writes about accepting difficulties, saying: "It's like inviting what scares us to introduce itself and hang around for a while."[2] I couldn't stand to hang around with what scared me. Who would? I was struggling mightily with how to dissolve the dualistic struggle. As the surgery date drew closer, I did my best to get by one day, and sometimes focusing on one hour at a time, without unraveling.

"I'm so proud of you!" Bonnie texted. "You are brave and strong."

"Freaking out," I wrote back. "I'm so scared."

Bonnie had researched The Surgery in much more depth than me. She suggested that I ask for a prescription of Xanax to help me stay calm. I remembered taking it once when I had an MRI. The stuff knocked me out. Maybe I could try a smaller dose. I happened to have a checkup with a psychiatrist coming up. When I got to the appointment, the woman at the front desk asked if it would be okay if a medical student observed. I said yes. I sat on a comfortable brown chair across from Dr. G. The medical student sat on a couch to my right. Dr. G asked how I was doing. I told her about my upcoming surgery and asked if she would prescribe Xanax because my anxiety was high. I started crying as I talked about it.

"You've made a very courageous decision," Dr. G said. That made me cry more. I didn't feel courageous.

"Thank you. It helps to hear that," I said. Tears poured down my face. I pulled some tissues out of the box next to me. Thankfully, her office always has plenty of tissues.

Once I got the pills, I decided to try one after work. I took half a pill and lay on the couch to watch TV. I couldn't stay awake. I texted Bonnie that it was making me too groggy.

"Your body will get used to it," Bonnie said. She was right. The next time I took it, I didn't feel as sleepy. Instead, it gave me some relief. At least temporarily.

I had made my decision. I wanted to go through with it. But the feeling of satisfaction I'd hoped for—that I'd be at peace with my decision and feel ready to boldly march forward like Angelina Jolie—well, it didn't come. Instead, I was terrified. I tried not to think about it. That did not work. Despite having this huge issue weighing on my mind, but I had a hard time talking about it. That feeling of embarrassment or maybe shame was still haunting me. It wasn't rational. I was afraid people wouldn't understand or they would feel like this was way too much information. Also, I didn't want people to feel sorry for me either. This kind of medical decision is such new territory. Tell people you've got cancer and they're immediately sympathetic and organizing meal deliveries. Tell them you're going to have a double mastectomy to prevent cancer and you may get a pause and that slow nod that means they're thinking "hmmmm . . . she seemed pretty normal until now."

The book *Confronting Hereditary Breast and Ovarian Cancer: Identify Your Risk, Understand Your Options, Change*

Your Destiny, advises readers not to let anyone change their mind about doing what's right for themselves. The book's authors, Sue Friedman, Dr. Rebecca Sutphen and Kathy Steligo wrote: "Gandhi said, 'I will not let anyone walk through my mind with their dirty feet,' and neither should you. This includes people who neither understand nor support your decisions. You're fortunate if everyone you encounter encourages your choices—that doesn't always happen. Not everyone will appreciate the risk you face or the challenge of making decisions when there are no great choices. Some people may question whether you're truly at high risk or may be of the impression that cancer can be cured, so why worry about it? No matter how close someone is to you, she can't possibly know what it's like to walk in your shoes unless she's had to make the same decisions."[3]

Some people simply don't know what to say.

"Sometimes people say nothing because they're afraid to say the wrong thing. At times, people say the wrong thing because they don't want to be silent. They want to support you; they just don't know how. Facing cancer risk or cancer itself is not the time to be stoic. It's a loving kindness to ask people for help and to let them know exactly what you need."

Eventually I told a few friends about my surgery. When I explained the situation and that I was thinking of surgery, a few said, "Wow, you really need to have this surgery." I had been seeing my boyfriend for only a few months. Telling someone you recently started dating that you're considering having a double mastectomy felt like a lot to bring into a new relationship. What if it was too much? I told him after we had lunch one day at a Thai place. I was nervous. I finally managed to explain that I have this high risk and that I've been struggling with the difficult decision to have this surgery.

"You mean like Angelina Jolie?"

"Yes, exactly." I explained the statistics and the options.

"You kind of have to do this," he said.

I told him about how awkward I felt since we hadn't been seeing each other that long. I didn't want it to affect anything.

"Leave me out of your decision," he said. He didn't get up and run out of the restaurant screaming. If he was freaked out about it, he didn't show it. We moved on to other topics and the whole ordeal wasn't nearly as bad as I had feared, as usual.

I received some responses that were more restrained, as if the person could not understand why I was having the surgery or did not think it was a good idea, or just didn't respond at all.

Most of all, I didn't want Leo, now nine, to be scared. There's a lot of advice for telling children about cancer but not so much about a probably someday cancer. I knew that just as important as what I told him was how I told him. If I seemed worried or upset, he would be too. I looked up information on FORCE about how to explain.

Some good tips on the FORCE site:

- Use simple, age-appropriate terms.
- Avoid premature reassurances and validate your child's concerns. Pushing a child's fears aside makes the situation appear too big and scary to talk about.
- Avoid unrealistic promises. Broken promises can diminish trust.
- Allow your child to tell you how little or how much she wants to know. Some children are more curious, others are more private.
- Allow your child age-appropriate participation in your process. Give him jobs to help him feel he is contributing.

I wanted him to know that I was having a surgery to keep me healthy and that I expected to be fine.

"I'm going to have a surgery soon. I'm not sick, but it's an operation to make sure I don't get sick," I said. I tried to keep a neutral tone that sounded like the surgery was not something to worry about. I explained that the doctors had to remove tissue from my breasts so that I could stay healthy. I explained that I'd stay home from work a while to recuperate, and that I may need him to help with certain jobs like lifting things.

He said okay and didn't seem upset or overly concerned. I asked if he had any questions. "You're not going to die, right?" he asked. He said it matter-of-fact, in a "I know this is true, but can you just confirm?" tone.

"No, sweetie," I said. "I've got the best doctors and they're going to take good care of me."

I hugged him, gave him a kiss and held him as long as I could before he squirmed away so he could go back to playing Minecraft.

Bonnie emailed me with some encouragement. She shared comments from the FORCE message board from women who had recently undergone PBMs and were doing well:

Patient 1: Awesome looking. I had an uneventful recovery as well. I was out walking in the neighborhood day 2 post op. I think a lot has to do with how your body is physically and nutritionally before surgery.

Patient 2: 6 weeks off, resting a LOT, taking it easy went back to work full time and the gym. Don't remember being tired when I went back to work. No complications at all. Not a lot of pain, I would describe it as pressure. Was off all pain meds after a week.

Patient 3: I had my exchange to 770cc Inspiras on 3–11–16 and honestly they already feel like a part of my body. I even catch myself lying on my stomach sometimes on the bed and it doesn't feel strange. I was a 38DDD before and now I'm a 38D so maybe they don't feel heavy to me because of my previous size though. Everyone is different.

Patient 4: I had my exchange almost 2 months ago. They already feel natural . . . for the most part I totally forget about em!

Patient 5: Two months out here and they feel like a part of me and have from day one! I kinda hated my old ones though—I appreciated them through nursing my babies, but I always knew in the back of my head they were going to kill me! Ever since I woke up from surgery, I have loved and appreciated my new ones. They may feel different occasionally, but they're a heck of a lot better than the old ones.

The week leading up to surgery was one of the most difficult of my life. I felt shockwaves of panic every day. I went to work, took Leo to school, shopped for groceries, cooked dinner, read with Leo at bedtime, all the normal day-to-day activities. Sometimes, I was able to stay in the moment. Others, my mind obsessed about the surgery. I was just trying to get through it.

I kept thinking: *Oh my God, am I really doing this?*

I went back to the conversations I had with my therapist.

"What are you afraid of?" she asked.

"Everything."

I had an appointment with Dr. E on the Monday before the surgery, which was scheduled that Friday. I checked in at the plastic surgery center. It's on the fifth floor of a large hospital medical center. Inside, it has stylish furniture and is filled with natural light from large windows. I walked past the brochures detailing facial rejuvenation, lipo and laser treatments and sat down in the waiting room and checked my phone.

"Kim," a nurse said a few minutes later.

I got up.

"How are you?" she asked.

"Okay," I lied.

My muscles were tight. I hadn't slept well in days. I could barely focus on anything. Someone led me to an exam room. As soon as I walked in I started bawling. I couldn't stop.

"Are you okay?" She headed toward the door, saying she was going to get the nurse.

"I'm okay. I'm just really nervous about the surgery." I grabbed tissues, wiped my eyes and blew my nose. I looked in the mirror. My eyes were red and swollen. I got more tissues.

The nurse came in. She sat down on a rolling stool and rolled over. She pulled in closer, looked me in the eye and talked in a low voice.

"If you don't want to do this, you don't have to. Just don't do it. Because you don't want to do this if your head isn't right about this. It's going to be hard."

She was giving me an out. I was not expecting that. Part of me wanted to get up and bolt out the door. I had permission to leave. Should I? I sat there, silent and staring at the floor, as these thoughts raced through my head.

The nurse continued.

"Wait till you get cancer. You don't know that you will but if you do, we'll catch it. Our guys are good."

I didn't want to "wait" for cancer. Suddenly, I felt the weight of not having the surgery. Of worrying about cancer, getting cancer and regretting not having the surgery. Oh no, I had worked too hard to get to this point. I had done my homework. I had climbed a mountain of fear and anxiety. No way was I turning back now.

I thought about why I was doing this. I pictured my son.

I shook my head.

"No, no. I'm okay. I've researched this carefully and I know I'm doing the right thing. I'm just scared. It's anxiety," I said, sobbing. "I'm okay."

She nodded. She squeezed my hand. "It'll be okay. We're going to take good care of you."

She told me to put on the pink gown I'd become so fond of. She left the room and a second later, Dr. E came in and sat on the stool in front of the computer.

"How are you?"

I had finally stopped crying. My eyes must have been red and puffy. I'm sure I looked fantastic.

"I'm okay. Just nervous about the surgery."

He was typing and looking at his screen.

"You gotta do it. That BRCA2 is just no good."

I nodded.

Dr. E had me sit on the exam table, which was a seat that could recline.

Dr. E studied my breasts. "The left one is slightly smaller." He made notes. I thought about how far I had come. A comment like that would have embarrassed me a few years ago.

"You're going to be fine. We'll make you look good."

I nodded. "Okay."

It still felt like we were talking about something in the abstract. It wasn't actually me having a double mastectomy, was it?

As the week went on, I stayed in won't-back-down mode. The idea of canceling the surgery made me more determined than ever. I had come too far. I tried to not think about the surgery but that was impossible. I tried to keep busy to ward off the flares of panic. Somehow, I got through the week. The Xanax helped. I took it Monday after work. It just made me sleepy. The next night, I decided to have a beer instead. Another night, it was a couple of glasses of wine. The goal was just getting through the week at that point. I worked through Wednesday, then created an out-of-office email before I left.

The day before the surgery, on Thursday, I had to spend half the day at the hospital undergoing tests and procedure called a lymphoscintigraphy to create a map of my sentinel lymph node, the first lymph node that would show a sign if cancer had spread. My surgeon recommended a sentinel node dissection, which means she would remove one lymph node for biopsy to make sure it was free of cancer. The procedure is a major improvement from previous generations, when all lymph nodes were taken during radical mastectomies, causing increased risk of infection and swelling. Not all surgeons do sentinel node dissections with a prophylactic bilateral mastectomy. Mine recommended it as a precaution.

The night before my surgery was the toughest. Leo was with his dad. I had asked him to record a video for me to watch when I was at the hospital. He made a sweet message about how I was going to be fine. My boyfriend came over and listened to me freak out. I drank a couple of glasses of wine. I thought of the John Lennon song "Whatever Gets You Thru the Night."

I wasn't allowed to have any food or drink after midnight. I was too wired to sleep. Finally, I was ready for bed. I set my alarm for 4 a.m. I had to leave for the hospital at 4:30 a.m.

The morning of my surgery, I watched the video my son made and looked at the picture of Angelina Jolie in a black evening gown that Bonnie had texted. The caption read: "Double Mastectomy? Double Badass!"

CHAPTER 8

The Angelina

"Above all, be the heroine of your life; not the victim."[1]

—Nora Ephron

May 20, 2016

Finally, Friday morning came. My mom picked me up at 4:30 a.m. We had to check into the hospital at 5 a.m. Surgery was at 7 a.m.

It was dark outside. We didn't talk much on the ride. I felt numb. The fact that this day that I had agonized about and dreaded for so long was here was a relief in a way. I had that sense as if, "Well shit this is really happening, isn't it?" I wasn't panicky. My body had given up on all its tantrums. Now, I was the stone-faced, blank-eyed inmate you see in movies being led into prison.

The waiting area was a wide-open place with several seating areas overlooking the first-floor lobby. Huge windows extended down to the floor below. All you could see was the night sky and the lights from the parking lot. Several people were already there. Everyone talked in low voices. It was too early for day-time volumes. I had a backpack with a few toiletries, a change of clothes, and books and magazines I didn't realize I would not have the concentration to read. My poor mom would have to carry the heavy black backpack around all day as I moved from pre-op to OR to recovery to hospital room.

We went up to the counter. The guy at the desk said he'd let them know I was there. A few minutes later, a woman called my name. We went into a small office facing the waiting area. It had a large screen she could slide closed for privacy.

What is your name?

Your date of birth?

What surgery are you having today?

I had to say it out loud. It was still hard to say the word.

We went through a list of questions. I got a plastic bracelet with my name and date of birth on it. I signed a bunch of forms acknowledging all the horrible things that could go wrong. I got a financial statement, an estimate of the cost of the surgery. The estimated cost that my insurance would allow for the surgery was $25,332.91. My portion, including a co-pay, deductible and co-insurance was an estimated $2,395.59. It was a huge amount for me, but I knew I was lucky because it could have been much worse.

Would I like to pay it all now?

Seriously?

Uh, no. I paid the least I could: half. I whipped out the handy credit card and signed the electronic pad to authorize $1,200. I had hoped to save enough money for the surgery but that didn't work out thanks to a never-ending stream of medical bills, co-pays and deductibles.

We sat back down in a waiting area. I was getting fidgety and uncomfortable. I couldn't focus. I was dying to get this thing started. I wanted to be knocked out ASAP. Pretty soon, a nurse led us to a pre-op room with a bed. It had three walls and a long curtain, which she closed. I answered more questions. The same questions. What is my name? What type of surgery am I having today? I changed into a lovely hospital gown and gave my bag of clothes to my mom, who sat on a chair next to me. There was a TV high up on the wall next to her. It wasn't on yet. All you could hear was doctors, nurses and other medical staff going by the curtain wall. I could not tell what they were saying. All I wanted to do was lie down and get hooked up to some medication that would knock me out. I asked if I could get something to help me relax. She said not yet. They had to do some tests and have me sign some documents. Someone took my temperature and blood pressure. The TV was turned on and the news was on, but I couldn't pay attention. I became more and more nervous, as various doctors, nurses and technicians came in and out. My heart was racing. I tried to breathe. All I wanted was for this to be over with. A woman finally came in to set up my IV. My muscles tensed. I wanted to be sedated.

After my IV was finished, a guy came in and asked if I wanted a nerve block. I didn't even know what that was. It was supposed to help reduce pain. I said yes.

My surgeon came in. She smiled, said good morning and shook my hand.

"We're going to take good care of you," she said.

"Thank you," I said.

Then Dr. E came in with an entourage of residents who looked like they could have all come off the *Grey's Anatomy* set. There were several guys in scrubs studying my breasts as I lay on the pre-op bed. They asked me to stand. I opened the gown. At one point, I had five doctors looking studiously at my breasts. Dr. R drew some marks on the top area of my breasts. Dr. E drew some. "Let's go here." "Can we go a little bit over?" It sounded like they were negotiating where to hang a picture. I was not shaking or trembling. At some point, you just accept the fact that you have become a canvas for their latest project. I stood there while the crew nodded and pointed and drew on my chest.

All I could think about was where were those drugs?

I remember a needle going into my shoulder or arm or somewhere. I remember hearing my mom talking about the pain she had suffered during a needle procedure. I couldn't wait for the drugs to work. That's the last thing I remember. I don't even remember being wheeled to the operating room.

It's strange to think of a team of surgeons and nurses working on you in the operating room. I was in the OR for nearly five hours. Just like after my hysterectomy, I have no memory of the recovery room. My mom said I cried like I did after my other surgery.

The day was a blur. I remember waking up in my hospital room and realizing that this was not a dream. My mom and Bonnie were there. It was afternoon and sunlight from the wall-length window filled the room. There were beautiful flowers from my mom and sister and a sweet care package from Bonnie—essentials such as wipes for the several days that I would not be able to shower and of course, chocolate. I was happy to see Bonnie, who was now living in New Mexico and had flown in to see me. We had promised to be there for each other's surgeries. I wasn't going to hold her to it. I know it's not easy to get away. It meant so much to see her there. I wasn't in pain, thanks to an IV. I was afraid to look under my hospital gown, but I pulled up the neck to peek. I couldn't see much under the bandages. The left side didn't look too much smaller than before. The other was flat. It looked like they let all the air out. The lack of breast tissue made a weird indention by my armpits. It was all so upsetting. I knew it was temporary, but I looked disfigured. I was so tired. Nothing seemed completely real. I drifted in and out of consciousness. Did this all really happen? I had flashes of freaking out and wondering if I had actually gone through with this. Eventually, I was starving. All they would let me eat was tasteless vegetable broth and some kind of overly sweet frozen thing. Later, I threw it all up like I did after my hysterectomy.

That night, I slept in spurts, waking up when nurses and techs came through on their rounds. I remember one of the techs being especially kind. The next day, a man came in with a tube I had to breathe into enough to move a ball to hit a certain number. Or something. I was zonked out most of the time.

Bonnie took a photo of my boobs. "You'll want this." I doubted that. They were completely bruised and bandaged. It looked awful.

Later, my ex said he would bring my son. There was a rule against anyone under age 12 visiting. I wanted to see him so badly. Could a nine-year-old pass? My ex said they'd try. It didn't work. My ex came in my room while my son stayed in the waiting area. I talked to him on the phone. He asked me how I was doing. After we hung up, I wanted to cry. My son was down the hall, in the waiting room. He was so close. And I couldn't see him.

I drifted in and out of sleep again that day. I could not sleep for long at any stretch, though, with nurses and techs coming in and out of the room. My boyfriend called to see how I was doing. I barely remember talking to him. I remember trying to check my email but forgetting my password to unlock my phone. I entered the wrong one so many times I disabled my phone. Later, I had to reset my phone and it wiped out my photos and videos, including the one Leo made for me that had been such a comfort before the surgery.

I woke up in the middle of the night on Saturday feeling the weight of everything that had happened. I was lying in the hospital bed and the tears started coming. I couldn't stop. The hugeness of the surgery was sinking in. Did I really do this? I could no longer waffle. It was done, and I couldn't go back. Tears kept running down the sides of my face.

A nurse came in for a routine check. She was tall, thin and pretty, with long blond hair. She was probably in her 40s. She asked what was wrong. I blubbered something between the tears about it being such a tough decision to have these mastectomies. She held my hand.

"You made the right decision," she said. "You are no less of a woman now." She said it in a kind, not condescending way, squeezing my hand. I cried even more after that. I felt so unbelievably sad. I don't know how much of it was an effect of the anesthesia and how much was from the impact of what I'd been through.

Finally, I fell asleep.

The next morning, I felt a lot better. I was going to my parents' house. I would get to see my son.

Before we could leave, the nurse showed me how to empty my drains. I had two thick plastic tubes, each about as wide as a straw, hanging out of the skin just below each armpit. The tubes came down past my waist. At the end, they were connected to small squishy oval bulbs that collected the blood and pus that continuously drained from my chest. I hated them. Each day, I'd need to squeeze all the blood out of each tube into the bulb and empty each bulb into a measuring cup. She gave us a sheet of paper with places for me to record my level of "output." I get queasy at the sight of blood. I was dreading having to empty these drains.

I wondered if Angelina Jolie felt the same way after her surgery. Jolie had hers at the Pink Lotus Breast Center in Beverly Hills, described on its website as an outpatient surgery center that provides an "attractive, peaceful alternative" to a hospital. I had an image in my mind of Angelina relaxing in a plush pink recliner, surrounded by flowers, while Brad Pitt (the surgery was before their divorce) attended to her every need. The part I couldn't imagine was Angelina Jolie with pus-filled drains hanging from under her arms.

CHAPTER 9

Surprise

"!@#$% Happens"[1]

 —Author Judy Blume, blogging about her breast
 cancer diagnosis

I stayed with my parents for several days after I got out of the hospital. My mom picked me up. The nurse brought me a wheelchair to get from my room to the lobby. The 30-minute drive to their home seemed like it took forever. Every slight bump was an earthquake. I felt nauseated. When I got to their house, I inched my way, as if I would detonate if I moved any faster, to the living room to plant myself on their comfy couch with a reclining seat that faces their flat-screen TV.

"You made a smart decision," my dad told me as I slowly raised the footrest.

"I feel like hell."

"Well, you were in a knife fight and you had no knife," he said.

My mom brought me a blanket.

I drifted in and out of sleep in my recliner and watched TV. I couldn't get enough of HGTV's magical healing properties. I binged on *Fixer Upper*, *House Hunters* and *Property Brothers*. Other than getting up to go to the bathroom and a few short and slow walks across the living room, I watched TV and slept for the first few days. I remembered the messages Bonnie sent about how well some women did after their mastectomies, including one who walked three miles three days after her surgery (or at least that's what I remember in the post-surgery haze). I could barely make it to the bathroom. I felt so fatigued, I couldn't imagine how anyone would bounce back so quickly after the surgery. The Pink Lotus center's website has a post by Angelina Jolie's surgeon saying that four days after surgery: "I was pleased to find her not only in good spirits with bountiful energy, but with two walls in her house covered with freshly assembled storyboards for the next project she is directing. All the while she spoke, six drains dangled from her chest, three on each side, fastened to an elastic belt around her waist."[2] Bountiful energy on Day Four? Freshly assembled storyboards? I could barely get to the toilet and reading a story, much less creating one, was out of the question. I was frustrated and sad that I felt so crappy. What was wrong with me? Unfortunately, painkillers, after-effects of anesthesia and the emotional toll of the surgery had hijacked my rational thinking skills, which would have reasoned that everybody recovers on their own schedule. Who knows if these women who seemed to be able to leap from surgery to marathon mall walks and work sessions had the same fitness level, general health and type of procedure. The Pink Lotus Breast Center website, for example, said that Angelina Jolie's sentinel lymph nodes were not removed. Mine were. Maybe that's part of why my energy wasn't as abundant. I was crazy to try to compare my progress to anyone else's. Then, after countless episodes of *Law & Order* and *Wheel of Fortune*, I was ready to take on another monumental task. I had to learn how to handle the dreaded drains. The drains were a big pain. They were stitched into the skin under each arm and taped down. The hospital had given me a plastic belt with Velcro straps and loops to hold the drain bulbs in place.

As if having four tubes hanging from under your arms, constantly draining blood and pus from where they removed all your breast tissue wasn't enough, the damn tubes jabbed me at their incision sites when I moved certain ways. It felt like I was being stabbed. The first time it happened, I yelled in pain. The only time it didn't hurt was if I walked with my arms out to my sides kind of like Frankenstein. My mom taped them in a way that kept them from moving as much. As I got over my squeamishness, emptying the drains became a daily ritual that broke up my sleeping, eating and watching TV routine. I didn't have the concentration to do much besides sleep and eat. Mostly, I didn't think too much about the surgery. Sometimes, I just cried, and I didn't know why.

Finally, about 10 days after my surgery, I switched to over-the-counter pain relief. I started to feel more like myself. I was allowed to take my first shower, with my mom standing outside the curtain just in case. I went to my own house, where I tried to focus enough to watch TV or read.

My friend Melissa came from Denver to take care of me for a few days after I went home. It was one of the kindest gifts I've ever received. Melissa, whom I've known since high school, went to the store on a Saturday morning and bought groceries then spent the rest of the day cooking as I drifted in and out of sleep. We talked, laughed and hung out. I slept. She cooked. We binge watched the hilarious Amazon comedy *Catastrophe*.

Leo stayed with his dad most of that weekend. I couldn't wait to have him back home and for life to get back to normal. My arms were still sore, and it was difficult to raise them enough to reach certain dishes or food in the pantry. The nurse told me not to lift anything heavier than a milk carton. I couldn't take out the trash. Leo helped me with chores like that and dealing with the litter box. We heated up the soup, chili, spanakopita and veggie burgers that Melissa had made.

A couple weeks after my surgery, it was time for a follow-up appointment with my breast surgeon.

I lay on the exam table and Dr. F checked my bruised, red breasts and said everything looked fine. Then she asked me to sit in a chair by her computer. She pulled up a report.

"There was a surprise in the pathology report," she said.

I smiled. All I heard was "pathology report." I was trying to get down from the exam table. She looked serious. Huh? I realized I had misunderstood. My heart started racing.

"The pathology found that you had DCIS," she said.

I looked at the screen. The pathology report said I had DCIS, ductal carcinoma in situ, in the right breast and atypical lobular hyperplasia in the left. DCIS is often called Stage 0 breast cancer. It's noninvasive, meaning that the abnormal cells have not spread outside the milk ducts. Atypical lobular hyperplasia is an abnormal growth that places people at higher risk of breast cancer.

I was in shock. My brain couldn't quite take it in. I had expected there might be some atypical cells since I'd had some before, but I wasn't expecting to hear that I had Stage 0 cancer.

I had spent so much time agonizing about whether to do the surgery. And here, a pathology report was saying that I did have cancer. I didn't—couldn't—say anything for a minute.

"I can't believe it."

"Your timing was excellent," Dr. F said.

The tumor was 4 mm, about the diameter of a birthday candle. It was ER-positive. And it was considered low nuclear grade, which means that it is less likely to come back after surgery.

Dr. F said the tumor was too small to show up on a mammogram. She said it may not have been identifiable on a mammogram for a year. I wonder though, if it was fast-growing like mom's, would it have become invasive quickly?

The news made me grateful and relieved that I had gone through with the surgery. I would not need any other treatment. No radiation. No chemo. I was done.

I felt incredibly lucky. After I got home, I needed to lie down. My boyfriend called. I told him the news.

"You should buy a lottery ticket," he said.

I wish I had.

Later, I cried the kind of tears that only come after an ordeal. My emotions ran the gamut. I was freaked out that there had been cancer in my body. I was grateful and relieved that it was gone. I was scared of what might have happened if I had not had the surgery. I was sad about all the time I spent agonizing and doubting. I thought about how I needed to try harder to make the most of and enjoy every moment of life. Then I drifted back to sleep.

Over the next several days, I gorged on information about DCIS. It was yet another confusing diagnosis to decipher. The significance of a DCIS diagnosis and the best treatment are subjects of ongoing debate. The issue is that some cases of DCIS may never become invasive, leading to concerns of overtreating the diagnosis. The problem is, science currently does not have a way to determine which DCIS tumors will become invasive and which ones will not. We just don't understand DCIS well enough yet.

DCIS accounts for about 20 percent of breast cancers, according to the American Cancer Society. DCIS rates increased dramatically after mammograms were introduced and helped detect much smaller tumors. Some in the medical community question whether DCIS should be called cancer at all and advocate taking the word "carcinoma" (the C in DCIS) out of the diagnosis. Apparently, I had the Rodney Dangerfield of breast cancers. My diagnosis went from a probably someday cancer to a kinda sorta cancer.

So did I have cancer or not? I searched various major cancer centers and breast cancer charities to find out how they described DCIS. Many organizations used the Big C word:

American Cancer Society: "DCIS is a non-invasive or pre-invasive breast cancer. This means the cells that line the ducts have changed to cancer cells but they have not spread through the walls of the ducts into the nearby breast tissue. Because DCIS hasn't spread into the breast tissue around it, it can't spread (metastasize) beyond the breast to other parts of the body. DCIS is considered a pre-cancer because sometimes it can become an invasive cancer. This means that over time, DCIS may spread out of the duct into nearby tissue, and could metastasize (spread). Right now, though, there's no good way to know for sure which will become invasive cancer and which ones won't. So almost all women with DCIS will be treated."[3]

Mayo Clinic: "Ductal carcinoma in situ (DCIS) is the presence of abnormal cells inside a milk duct in the breast. DCIS is considered the earliest form of breast cancer. DCIS is non-invasive, meaning it hasn't spread out of the milk duct and has a low risk of becoming invasive."[4]

Susan G. Komen: "DCIS (ductal carcinoma in situ) is a non-invasive breast cancer. In DCIS, the abnormal cells are contained in the milk ducts (canals that carry milk from the lobules to the nipple openings during breastfeeding). It's called "in situ" (which means "in place") because the cells have not left the milk ducts to invade nearby breast tissue. DCIS is also called intraductal (within the milk ducts) carcinoma. You may hear the terms "pre-invasive" or "pre-cancerous" to describe DCIS. DCIS is treated to try to prevent the development of invasive breast cancer."[5]

JohnsHopkins Medicine: "Ductal Carcinoma in Situ (DCIS) is non-invasive breast cancer. Because it is limited to being inside the duct of the breast, it is classified as being Stage 0."[6]

Call it whatever you want. I was just glad it was gone.

CHAPTER 10

From A to B

"You can get better boobs than you had before, if you so choose."[1]

—Christina Applegate, breast cancer survivor and BRCA1 mutation carrier

Nora Ephron felt bad about her neck. I felt bad about my upper chest area. I had oval concave areas above each breast where breast tissue was removed. In a preventative mastectomy, the breast surgeon removes as much breast tissue as possible. Breast tissue, it turns out, goes much higher than the actual breast. The mastectomy left a shallow hollowed-out area that goes nearly up to my collarbone. It looked as though someone took a big spoon and pressed it into my chest area above each breast. I worried that I'll never feel confident about wearing a tank top or shirt with a collar lower than a crew neck.

The best I could hope for is that a procedure called fat grafting could help fill in that area. That's where they take fat from your stomach (thankfully I had plenty for this purpose) and use it to fill in the chest area. They do this when they take out the expanders and put in your implants.

I asked Dr. E about it.

"Can I get fat grafting?"

He hesitated.

"We can *try* it," he said, looking doubtful.

"You don't sound too optimistic," I said.

Dr. E said the problem is that the fat doesn't always stay in place. Dr. E said he would give it a try though. I figured it couldn't hurt. For now, we were focused on expanding my skin to make space for the implants. Dr. E had put in expanders after the breast surgeon did the mastectomy. I would go to his office on my lunch hour every couple of weeks to have more saline injected into them. The expanders were cool. They had an injection site with a self-sealing port and guard to prevent the needle from puncturing the implant during injections. The nurse used a locator that had a magnet to find the port.

My days were a blur of lying around, sleeping and watching TV, hanging out with my son and a few visits from my boyfriend, family members and friends. One day my big outing was to a thrift store to buy a long button-down shirt. These had become my new uniform. I wore leggings, a tank top and a large button-down shirt every day during my recovery. The main reason was because I couldn't raise my arms to put on a T-shirt. Bonnie had read so much about surviving the surgery, she taught me the trick of putting on tank tops by pulling them up from my legs. My favorite outfit was black leggings, a black tank top and a light button-down shirt with a large black and white plaid design. The baggy button-down shirts were functional—they did a great job of covering my drainage bulb tool belt. Although they hid the blood- and pus-filled bulbs, they bulged out on each side, making it look like I had a condition where an unnatural amount of body fat had accumulated on the sides of my hips. When you're recovering and not feeling well, you don't even care.

Three weeks after my surgery, my daily drain output was hovering around 30 ml, enough to fill a shot glass. I was so close. I called Dr. E's office and told one of the nurses about my progress. It was a Friday. I got excited thinking about the prospect of not having to go through the weekend being stabbed and sore.

The nurse wasn't as impressed.

"Let's see how they do over the weekend."

What a letdown.

"Okay. I guess I was just over-eager," I said. "I hate these things."

She was sympathetic.

"I know. Everyone wants those out. But you don't want to get a seroma. You want to make sure to leave them in long enough." A seroma is a pocket of fluid that can lead to swelling and possibly infection.

Finally, the following week, my output dropped to 20 ml per drain. This was big.

I called Dr. E's office.

The nurse said I could come in the next day. I set an appointment for 10:30 a.m., the earliest available. I could not wait.

By this point, I could drive. I tried not to speed on the way to Dr. E's office.

They called me back after a few minutes in the waiting room. In the exam room, I put on my gown as usual and waited in the exam chair.

A nurse came in.

"How are you doing? Ready to get those drains out?"

"Yes. I am soooo excited."

"It's the little things, right?"

I sat on the exam table and took my arm out of the left side of my gown. The nurse came toward me with a metal tool. I couldn't look. I turned my head in the other direction. I felt a tug as she plucked out the stitches that kept the tube in place. I peeked. Next, she was pulling a long tube out from the hole under my armpit. Inside, the tube wound through my entire chest. The whole thing may have only lasted several seconds but it felt like my veins were being yanked out. I gripped the hard vinyl seat cushion. She cleaned and bandaged the area. It was so sore, I couldn't put my arm down along my side any better than when the tube was in.

I watched her throw the bloody bandaging, tube and drain bulbs in the trash. She did the same thing on the right side. Then she bandaged it up.

Then I got ready for another fill.

Dr. E came in.

"Looking good. How much are we doing today?"

He settled on 100 cc in just the left. I've been asked how big I plan to go. One of the biggest regrets some women post on the FORCE boards is that they didn't go bigger. I'm not interested in being much bigger. I'll go to a small B.

The nurse went to the counter to get the gadget that uses a magnet to find the port, so she could stick in the needle.

I couldn't look. I turned to the right and focused on a wall of brochures. Liposuction. Chin lift. Tummy tuck. I squeezed the seat cushion.

"Alright, you're done," Dr. E said.

I barely felt it.

"Really? I was bracing myself."

Some of the blogs and message boards I've read say that the fills put so much pressure on the skin, they hurt. Luckily, mine didn't.

A few weeks after my surgery, I felt ready to tackle the gym. I signed up for a membership at the rec center near my house. I rode a stationary bike slowly for 30 minutes. I became a regular.

My medical leave lasted eight weeks. On the last week, I had to get a note from my doctor letting my employer know that I was able to come back to work. It was early July. On that first Monday when I went back to the office, the first thing I needed to do was take my doctor's note to the human resources department. I read it one last time. Under the question "reason for medical leave" on the form, my doctor wrote "breast cancer." Reading the form was a little jarring, as if seeing the words in print made it sink in a bit more that I had cancer. My hands shook as I gave it to the person in the HR office.

That summer, I went in about once every two weeks for a "fill." I tried to arrange the appointments during my lunch break. The nurses usually did the fills. On one day, it was a nurse I hadn't met before.

I was in my gown, sitting on the examination table as casually and routinely as if I was going for coffee at Starbucks.

The nurse asked me to open my gown. By this time, I wasn't fazed. Somehow, I was less shy about showing my foobs than I was about the real ones.

"You look GOOD," she said. "They did a great job."

"Thanks!" I said.

I had started to like how the expanders looked and was getting a little worried about whether I'd like the implants as much. The nurse told me about one patient who kept her expanders in for years.

In August, I had an appointment with Dr. E. He looked at my charts to see how much saline had been injected into my expanders. He said I'd be ready for my exchange surgery soon. Much sooner than I expected. I'd read that the expander process can take six months. It had only been two and a half months since my surgery. Dr. E said we could schedule the surgery in six weeks, which would mean I had the expanders for four months.

We set a date for the surgery on Sept. 16, 2016.

Every time I made it over another decision hurdle, I landed in front of another one. This time, I had to choose a type of implant. Implants come in different shapes and can be filled with either silicone or saline. The decision, like everything else, is complicated.

First, did I want silicone or saline? I liked the idea of saline because it seemed less toxic than silicone. I had interviewed women suffering from health problems due to leaking silicone implants for a paper I worked at in the 1990s. Their class-action lawsuit against the implant manufacturers led to an FDA moratorium on all silicone implants in 1992. The FDA lifted the moratorium in 2006, opening the way for a new generation of silicone implants. My doctors said the newer implants were safe. The silicone was in a thick gel, rather than a liquid form, that is not supposed to leak if it ruptures. They even had a cute name: "gummy bear" implants. Saline implants, on the other hand, were filled with saline water. They feel harder than a silicone implant. If a saline implant ruptured, saline would leak into your body rather than silicone. But since saline is essentially as thin as water, if it ruptures, the implant goes completely flat. You could be on a date, giving a presentation at work, teaching a class, or whatever, and suddenly one of your breasts goes from a D to less than an A as the water gushes out of it and into your body.

Dr. E recommended silicone. I had mixed feelings. After doing some research, I decided to go with silicone.

That led to the next question: Round or teardrop-shaped implants?

"I don't know. What do you recommend?" I asked Dr. E. "Which would be best to fill in this area?"

I pointed to the hollowed area above my breasts.

Dr. E stared at my chest studiously. By this time, I had gotten used to the clinical ogling.

"I think a teardrop implant will be best for filling in that area," he said. "The only thing is, teardrop implants can turn sideways. It happens maybe 15 percent of the time. If it happens, it requires another surgery."

Sometimes we hear what we want or need to hear. I focused on the part about it covering more of my concave area and less on the part about needing an additional surgery.

I asked what it would look like if the implant went sideways. He showed me a photo of a woman who had one normal-looking breast and one that was too misshapen to cover up by throwing on a cardigan.

"You would do surgery to fix it if that happened?" I asked for reassurance.

"Yes. But you can't do the surgery until at least three months after the implant initially was placed there," he said.

So, I would have to go around for a few months, potentially, with a weird sideways boob that would be hard to hide? Can't anything with this BRCA stuff be simple?

"Well, I still think I'd like to try the teardrop implant if you think that's going to give me the best result," I said. "How long should I expect to take off work?"

"I'll do the surgery on a Friday. A lot of patients are back to work on Monday or Tuesday."

That was encouraging. This would be easier than I expected. I had thought I would need to wait until November or December.

It would be nice to get this over with before the holidays.

I told my boss I'd need time off and filled out paperwork with HR. The note from the doctor's office said I should be cleared for up to two weeks off. I asked the nurse about that.

"Why? What did Dr. E tell you?"

"He said I could go back to work on Monday or Tuesday," I said.

"You'll need more than that. I would take off at least a week," she said.

After the mastectomies, I thought the exchange surgery would be a breeze. I wasn't nearly as nervous as before the mastectomy.

Once again, my mom picked me up. We had to arrive at the hospital at 7:30 a.m.

We checked in. I had to put $1,000 on my credit card. I was going broke.

I went through a lot of the same drill as with the last surgery. I was becoming a pro. In the pre-surgery room, I changed into my gown and lay down on the hospital bed. The anesthesiologist introduced himself, asked a few questions and left.

A nurse checked my temperature, pulse, etc. Then she tried to set up the IV. I was lying there, eager for anesthesia time. She was having trouble with the IV. My veins were "rolling." She seemed frustrated. I got nervous. Another nurse came in and appeared to have the same trouble. It was unnerving to have them poking at you over and over.

All the while, my Mom talked to me to try to keep me calm. It didn't work. She played a video of my nephew performing in a play. I couldn't see well. I couldn't focus. She was holding up the phone with video while the nurse was poking my veins. I just wanted someone to put me under. Nurse finally got a vein and set up IV. I hoped for drugs ASAP.

The nurse said they were waiting for Dr. E to finish his first surgery. Not much later, Dr. E came in. He said he just operated on someone whose teardrop implant had turned sideways.

"What kind of implant are we doing?" he asked.

"Didn't we decide on teardrop?" I said. "Please go with the one you think is best."

"Okay. I'll try each kind to see what looks best. I'll have the women in the OR give their opinions," Dr. E said.

"Okay, thanks," I said. "And you're going to do fat-grafting, too?"

Dr. E said he would.

I couldn't wait to get started. Waiting in the pre-surgery room has got to be one of the worst types of waiting.

Last thing I remember is them saying Dr. E was ready for me.

I woke up later in the recovery room.

I alternated between not being able to keep my eyes open and feeling uncharacteristically chatty.

Dr. E visited. I remember saying I have two questions.

"Is it okay to use arnica?" This is a homeopathic medication that my friend told me Angelina Jolie used. It's for bruising and swelling. If Angelina used it, I wanted it too.

"You can try it, but I wouldn't buy it if it's expensive," Dr. E said.

I'd heard that a high fat diet is recommended after fat grafting so that the body doesn't burn the fat that has been placed in the breasts. I asked Dr. E if eating a high-fat diet will help prevent the fat from being reabsorbed. He looked at my mom. Then at me—as if I was insane. I don't remember his answer. My mom had a good laugh over that idea.

Exchange surgeries are an outpatient procedure. It's a little unnerving to go home all bandaged up, with drains hanging out of your body and feeling barely coherent. It didn't feel like I should be out of the hospital. All I remember is going to my parents' house and falling asleep.

The next day, I mostly slept and watched TV. My mom, dad and I blew through *The Killing*, a great detective series on Netflix. My dad made his famous grilled cheese and fries.

I emptied my drains. I took painkillers. This was getting to be a way too familiar routine. Detectives Holder and Linden finally got together. I was so happy. The pain medication was working.

On Monday, I had a follow-up appointment with Dr. E.

The nurse asked for my logs. I didn't keep any this time. Dr. E had said I only needed the drains over the weekend.

"I can't remove these. I don't think they're ready. You don't want to get a seroma," she said.

No, no, NO, I thought. Hopefully this was a mistake.

"I'm sorry. I may be confused but my mom said Dr. E said to come back on Monday and he'd take them out."

The nurse left the room and came back a few minutes later.

"I just saw Dr. E. He said they were just supposed to stay in for the weekend. So, I'll take them out."

"Phew."

Amy stood on my right side and started to take the tape off my skin surrounding the area where the tube was stitched in. I looked away. I felt some tugging as she cut the stitches that held in the tube.

"Okay, dear. Take a deep breath."

I tried my best as my heart pounded.

"Now, slowly release your breath."

As I did, I felt a pulling as if she was slowly and gently yanking an endless string from my insides. I gripped the seat with my left hand and squeezed my eyes shut.

"I'm sorry."

"It's okay," I said. "It's such a weird feeling."

Next, she did the other side.

The next day, I felt down. Coming off the anesthesia can do that, but at the time, you don't realize it could be the medication. I looked at my chest and saw bandages, bruises and swelling. I was exhausted. What about these stories I'd heard on the message boards of the exchange surgery being such a breeze?

A few days after the surgery, I felt incredibly fatigued. I hurt. I had a constellation of small bruises on my thighs, my butt and in several spots on my stomach from the fat grafting procedure. It looked like I had been beat up by a bunch of my son's mini-figures.

Technically called autologous fat transfer, in fat grafting plastic surgeons use a thin tube to suck fat from one area and inject it into the chest.

I did not prepare myself for it to hurt like hell. I was sore and bloated. I was tired of hurting. I felt a little sorry for myself and then felt guilty. I thought about how difficult it must be for people who have gone through chemo. I knew I was lucky. At the same time, I was in a lot of pain.

I had some time on my hands, so I decided to watch some shows I'd never gotten around to seeing. I watched several episodes of *The Wire* but it was depressing. I tried *Breaking Bad*. That was even more depressing. I needed something light. I was worried about being off work. I had no reason to worry. I was fortunate to have a great job and understanding supervisors. Anxiety was taking over. As usual, it snuck up on me and I didn't see it for what it was. I worried about everything that anxiety could find to worry about. I worried about my implants. I worried that my teardrop implant would flip sideways. I read online about cases in which that happened. I started second guessing myself. Should I not have had teardrop implants? What if it flips? After all this pain, I didn't want another surgery ever again. How could I prevent it from flipping? I googled around but didn't find much advice. The clearest thing I could find was that the possibility of it flipping could depend on whether the surgeon was able to fit the implant tightly into a pocket.

Once the bruises healed, I noticed something. My breasts looked good.

A couple weeks after the exchange surgery, I had another follow-up appointment. Once again, I took the elevator to the fifth floor. The nurse took me back to the examination room.

Gown open to the front. I looked at myself in the full-length mirror. Another nurse came in to take my blood pressure.

"Dr. E has a resident with him today. Is it okay if he brings him?"

"Sure."

I change into the gown and sit on the chair. They come in after a couple minutes. Dr. E introduces me to the resident, a young, good-looking guy.

"Let's take a look," Dr. E. said.

I open the gown.

Dr. E. stands there, looking at my chest and nodding.

"It looks really good," he said to the resident, who nodded back at him.

Dr. E told the resident he used a teardrop implant and fat grafting. He said if the fat stays after three months, it should stay long-term. He said if the implant flips sideways, he'll come back in and put in round implants that I can keep for the rest of my life.

I asked if I can exercise yet.

"What type of exercise do you want to do?"

"Running."

"That's fine."

"Cycling."

"That's fine."

"Yoga."

"No. you need to give the muscles time to heal. You can do yoga in December."

Dr. E said to come back in three months. I left overjoyed at the thought of three whole months without a doctor's appointment.

I didn't make it that long.

The next month I felt pain and soreness in my left breast. It hurt to move my left arm and I could barely raise it. I was convinced I had an infection. I googled around and became concerned I had a capsular contraction, a complication that develops when scar tissue surrounds and constricts the implant. Even worse, I worried it could be cancer.

I made an appointment with Dr. E.

"It's not an infection," he said.

I was surprised.

"It's a fat necrosis," he said. "We can scan it, but I know that's what it is."

A fat necrosis. Why does everything have to sound so gross. I looked it up. It's just dead fat. Some of the fat injected from my butt, stomach or thigh probably had hardened.

Dr. E ordered an ultrasound as a precaution. The results did not rule out a problem.

The report stated:

> There is an oval heterogeneous solid mass with circumscribed margins and parallel orientation measuring 12 x 5 x 10 mm seen in the right reconstructed breast at 3 o'clock located 1 centimeter from the nipple. No blood flow is detected within the lesion on Doppler analysis. This finding corresponds to the area of palpable concern.

Next, I would need a biopsy. I was scared. Could it be more than a necrosis? It would be rare to have a tumor, especially right after my surgery. Could they have missed some of the cancer? I thought about how awful it would be to go through preventative surgery and still get cancer. I was so sick of medical appointments. I was burning through what little sick time I had built up since my surgery.

I went to my appointment for the biopsy. I lay on an exam table. The doctor was going to stick a needle in the area to get a tissue sample. I started to worry it could puncture the implant.

There was an ultrasound guiding the process. The chances were slim, according to the doctor. If it did, how would I know? She said I'd see swelling and redness.

The doctor cleaned the area. I couldn't feel anything on my skin. I felt a sensation of the needle when she gave me a local anesthetic. She asked me about my surgery. I explained that I had the mastectomy and implants because I have a BRCA2 mutation. I said I had spent years agonizing over whether to have the surgery. And I told her that when I finally had the surgery, the pathology showed that I had DCIS.

"That gives me chills," she said. "Sometimes you just know. Your body knows."

The biopsy came back benign, a huge relief.

I was still sore. It still hurt to raise my left arm. What was going on?

Dr. E said it's not uncommon for women to have soreness after a mastectomy. He referred me to a physical therapist who specialized in helping women who have had mastectomies. I didn't want to miss any more work. I scheduled an appointment as close to my lunch break as possible to minimize sick time.

The physical therapist worked out of the same office as my breast surgeon and oncologist. She had me lie on my back on the table. There were a few pieces of exercise equipment and a bookshelf with a lot of books about cancer.

She had me move my arms up and down and to the side to measure and record my range of motion. Next, she pressed her hands into the long thick scars under my breasts to break up scar tissue. The "massage" hurt like hell. My face tightened as she dug into those scars and I gripped the side of the massage table. Tears streamed from my eyes. Somehow, though, I felt so much better afterward. Arm stretches came next. My poor arms had been babied too much and maybe that had caused the soreness in the first place. After a few sessions, my arms felt back to normal.

At a follow-up appointment with Dr. E, I told him about how well the physical therapy worked. I mentioned that my scars itched a lot.

He said he could give me steroid shots. It would make a big difference.

"Okay," I said, willing to try anything.

Dr. E left the room and came back with a needle. He stuck it into my scar under my left breast. It stung with sharp pain. He quickly stuck it in a few other places along the scar. Holding my breath, I tensed up and gripped the exam table seat. It hurt, then it was over. This may have been a case of the treatment causing more pain than the problem.

"Come back in a month and we can see if you need more," he said.

After I made the appointment, I wondered why I was signing up for more pain. I called later to cancel it. The scars were okay as far as I was concerned. Over time, the scars stopped itching so much, though they flare up now and then. The raised, red lines look and feel like al dente spaghetti noodles running underneath my breasts.

Once I got past the fat necrosis, the post-surgery tenderness and the muscle pain, life started to get back to normal. My implants felt okay, but not like real breasts. They aren't as soft. They have little sensation. (Doctors warn you not to use a heating pad near them because you won't feel it and some women have burned their skin that way.) They barely squish when you hug someone or lie on your stomach. They don't move when you run or jump. Like anything, there are good things that come with the not so good. On the plus side, you don't need to wear a bra if you don't want to. They even make stick-on "petals" you can put over your nipples if you're concerned about them showing. Best of all, these babies will never sag. They don't feel like foreign objects in my body. I barely noticed or thought about them after a while. As for the concave areas above my breasts, they were still there. Not as bad as before, but still there. The fat grafting may have helped smooth over the area a little. I don't know if it was worth it. But overall, Christina Applegate was right: you really can get better-looking boobs than you had before.

CHAPTER 11

It's Always Something

"Life is about not knowing, having to change, taking the moment and making the best of it, without knowing what's going to happen next."[1]

> —Gilda Radner, who died in 1989 at age 42 from ovarian cancer

June 2018

I don't have cancer. Nearly 10 years after I took the risk assessment that started this whole BRCA2 saga, I am sitting in a doctor's office for the umpteenth time. This time, it's for a simple routine checkup with the breast surgeon. The person at the desk gave me several pages of forms to fill out with a long list of conditions and symptoms. I had to check yes or no boxes by each one. Some sounded scary: sudden weight loss, loss of appetite or sense of smell or taste. The waiting room has a large wall of windows looking out to a gorgeous clear blue sky, HGTV playing at a low volume on the TV across the room of neatly arranged chairs. Before I could figure out which show it was, the nurse called my name. She led me down the hall to get my weight and blood pressure. Then she took me to an exam room and handed me the pink gown with little dark pink swirls and snaps in the front. Undress from the top, open to the front. I sat waiting, reading the day's depressing news on my phone.

From now on, I will have regular appointments like this one to check for any signs of cancer. There's nothing else I can possibly have removed from my body to lower my cancer risk. The coding error in my genes could still cause a cancer to develop. I could get another breast cancer, though my risk is now lower than that of the average woman. Having a BRCA2 mutation means I still have higher-than-average risks for a few other cancers, including pancreatic and melanoma. And although my ovaries are gone, I still have a small but elevated risk of peritoneal cancer, a rare type that involves tissue in the stomach cavity lining. As Gilda Radner's famous SNL character, Roseanne Roseannadanna used to say: "It's always something. If it's not one thing it's another."

I will continue seeing a team of specialists. There's the breast surgeon, oncologist, gynecological oncologist, gastroenterologist and the dermatologist. The dermatologist is the easiest part. I make an appointment once a year. I have fair skin, a lot of freckles. I burn easily and had more than a few serious sunburns when I was a kid, so having a higher risk of a melanoma because of the BRCA2 mutation is scary. At least you can be screened by a dermatologist to check for any signs of cancer.

Peritoneal and pancreatic cancers are a different story. There are no reliable tests to screen for early signs of either. At my annual appointment with my gynecological oncologist, the doctor checks me by pressing gently into different parts of my pelvic area. I hope if something ever goes wrong, he will be able to feel it. Otherwise, symptoms could be vague, such as bloating or a feeling of fullness, like with ovarian cancer. A woman at a local FORCE meeting told the group she found out she had peritoneal cancer after becoming concerned about bloating that made her skirts really tight around her waist. My doctors tell me not to worry about peritoneal cancer because it's so rare. Of course, any time I feel bloated, that's where my mind goes.

My oncologist recommended I see a gastroenterologist who is working on a study using MRIs to screen for early signs of pancreatic cancer. Pancreatic cancer is not common—it affects only 1 percent to 2 percent of people in the general population. However, the risk rises to 5 percent in people with BRCA mutations.[2] I keep picturing myself in a room of 100 people with BRCA2 mutations. Five of us will get it at some point in our lives, if the statistic is accurate. Pancreatic cancer is usually caught late because there are often no obvious signs in the early stages. Symptoms—abdominal or back pain, weight loss, jaundice (yellowing of the skin and eyes), loss of appetite, nausea, dark colored urine, changes in stool or appetite—can be vague and easily attributed to other things. Three out of four patients die within a year of diagnosis. Fewer than one in 10 survive more than five years.[3] Pancreatic cancer has the highest mortality rate of all major cancers. The American Cancer Society estimated that 55,440 people will be diagnosed with pancreatic cancer in a year and 44,330 people would die of the disease in 2018.[4]

As much as I wanted to participate in the pancreatic cancer screening test, I worried about the potential effects of having so many MRIs. The U.S. Food and Drug Administration (FDA) issued a "safety announcement"[5] in July 2015 that it was investigating the risk of brain deposits following repeated use of gadolinium-based contrast agents (GBCAs) for MRIs. It is unknown whether these gadolinium deposits are harmful. I felt another wave of panic when I found out about the possible long-term consequences of the screenings designed to protect me from cancer. By that point, I'd already had a bunch of breast MRIs using the contrast. Who knows how much gadolinium could be hanging out in my body. The Radiology Society of North America issued a press release[6] saying that research in the journal

Radiology suggests that some types of the contrast agent may remain in the brain for years, but that the long-term effects are unknown. FORCE also posted information about the research[7] on its website, saying that experts on its advisory board believe that the known benefits outweigh the theoretical risk.

I made an appointment with the gastroenterologist. I told her I wanted to enroll in the study, but I was concerned about the long-term effect of gadolinium. She said we could do the MRIs without contrast, but they would not work as well. I decided to go ahead with a regular MRI. Having the screening brought back worries about the possibility of another series of follow ups, biopsies and false alarms or worse. I took off an afternoon from work to go to the outpatient center by the hospital. Unlike breast MRIs, you lie on your back for the pancreatic cancer screening. I slid into the narrow tube and after a lot of loud beeps and video game battle sounds, it was over. The test revealed that my pancreas was fine.

The MRI and checkups gave me a sense of comfort that I had a plan to check on my health going forward. There wasn't much more I could do except try not to worry about cancer and go "live my life," as my breast surgeon advised after my surgeries.

I was working on that when I learned about yet another type of cancer that sort of threw me over the edge. The warning came six months after my exchange surgery in a *New York Times* headline: "A shocking diagnosis: Breast implants gave me cancer."[8] The article was about a woman who had breast implants after reconstructive surgery following a cancer diagnosis. After fighting breast cancer and going through chemo, she was diagnosed years later with a rare cancer called breast implant-associated anaplastic large-cell lymphoma (also referred to as BIA-ALCL), which has been linked to certain implants. Most cases involved implants with a textured, rather than smooth, surface. My stomach was in double knots as I read. Were those the same kind of implants that I have? When I got home, I checked the manufacturer information on my implants. They were Naturelle and, just my luck, they were textured. If I had known about this risk, I wouldn't have chosen this type of implant. Had I not done enough homework? I thought I'd researched all this stuff to death. When I Googled anaplastic large-cell lymphoma, I realized that the information available before 2017 was limited and vague. One message board entry on the topic said the odds were two in 1 million. In early 2017, several months after my exchange surgery, the U.S. Food and Drug Administration posted information that it had received more than 300 medical device reports of BIA-ALCL, including nine deaths. A September 2017 update[9] states that the FDA has received 414 medical device reports of implant-associated anaplastic large-cell lymphoma so far. Of the reports, 272 cases included information about the type of implant surface. Most, or 242 implants, had textured surfaces, while 30 had smooth surfaces. A little more than half, 234, were silicone, while 179 were filled with saline. After all I'd gone through, I'd be outraged and devastated if I made the wrenching decision to go through my surgeries only to get cancer from my implants. I talked to my breast surgeon about it. I pulled up a copy of the article on my phone. She knew about the news reports. She said she understood my concern. But she emphasized that the risk of that happening is extremely low, about 1 in 30,000.

"You're more at risk getting on the highway," she said.

The doctor added that anaplastic large-cell lymphoma was highly treatable.

"What symptoms would I look for?" I asked.

"Redness and swelling," she said.

I wanted to cry. I was so frustrated to discover that I could get cancer from the damn implants. My breast surgeon said she didn't recommend having surgery to replace them since the risk was so tiny. My anxiety had found something new to grab onto and would not let go. Why did this bother me so much? Why did this particular risk, the smallest by far of all the cancer risks I face, stick in my brain, as if all my prevention efforts were ruined? Was I really so afraid of this miniscule risk—or did it bother me so much because it made me realize how little control, beyond having my surgeries, screenings and checkups, I truly have?

The risk from my breast implants, small as it was, forced me to face the fact that there was only so much I could do to prevent cancer. After having my ovaries, fallopian tubes and breast tissue removed, all I could do was to have regular checks and screenings and live a healthy lifestyle. Beyond that, well, what can you do but make the best of it?

After a few minutes of waiting in the exam room, I heard a light knock on the door.

The nurse practitioner came in.

"How are you doing?" she asked.

"Pretty good."

She motioned for me to sit on the exam table.

"Do you have any concerns?"

"Not really, everything feels pretty normal," I said.

The nurse practitioner did a clinical exam, feeling the surface of my breasts and gently pushing into my pelvic area.

"Everything looks great," she said. "Do you have any questions?"

After years of questions, I've practically run out.

"You're doing well," she said. "We'll see you back in a year."

I made an appointment for a year later and said goodbye to the scheduler. As I walked through the cancer center lobby and passed other patients, I thought about how different things could have turned out if I had not had my surgeries when I did. I'm nine years older now than grandmother was when she died of breast cancer. And thanks to my double mastectomy, I don't have to worry anymore that I probably will get breast cancer. Even though I still have risks, The Surgery gave me the peace of mind of knowing that I have done everything I can to lower my odds of cancer. Despite all my anxiety and fear leading up to that decision, life after the surgery didn't feel so different from life before surgery. The Surgery I dreaded so much seemed more like the surgery to me. I could even say the word mastectomy. I felt extremely lucky to be leaving the cancer center without having to worry about going back for another MRI or biopsy. Life was back to normal.

I got in my car and headed back to work. Later, I would pick up my son from school. We needed to stop at the grocery store. Maybe we'd get pizza for dinner. Then I would do a load of laundry. My to-do list raced through my mind as the cancer center disappeared from my rearview mirror.

Epilogue

My mom, sister and I were the first ones in our family to discover that we inherited the harmful BRCA2 mutation 8803delC.

Now that we've been tested, what about the next generation?

My sister who has a BRCA mutation and I each have one son. Each has a 50–50 chance of inheriting the mutation from us. I'd give anything for them to be spared so the mutation would end with my sister and me. (We have another sister who did not test positive for the mutation so her three children thankfully are not at risk.)

When my son, Leo, is grown up, I will encourage him to get tested. Genetic counselors suggest waiting until age 18 at the earliest. If he has the harmful mutation, his breast cancer risk thankfully would be very low, but higher than that of the average man. He also would face an increased risk of prostate cancer and pancreatic cancer and, if he has children, especially daughters, he could pass it on to them. By that time, I hope that there will be better solutions for dealing with BRCA mutations.

We also are finding out about more positive tests for BRCA2 mutations in our extended family. In 2018, my cousin on my mom's side went through genetic testing and discovered that she has the same mutation. She has found a physician with expertise in BRCA issues and decided to go forward with a double mastectomy and bilateral salpingo-oophorectomy. She has two children: a son and a daughter.

Our options for preventing BRCA-related cancers are limited right now. But at least we can do something. If only my grandmother, Lucy Belle, great-grandmother, Margaret, and great-great aunts who died so young had had that chance. Before BRCA mutations were identified, women like Lucy Belle and Margaret had to deal with their risk in fear and darkness. We may not be able to remove the threat from our genes (yet), but we can try to prevent cancer from cutting more lives short. For the first time in history, we've got a shot at turning a probably someday cancer into a probably never cancer.

Acknowledgments

I owe thanks to so many people. Thank you to the Mayborn Literary Nonfiction Conference manuscript competition judges for selecting my manuscript. Thank you to the University of North Texas Press in Denton for publishing this book. I am indebted to Ron Chrisman, Director, and Karen DeVinney, Managing Editor, for their excellent advice and editing. I appreciate the anonymous reviewers who gave their time to read my manuscript and provide invaluable feedback. Thanks also to the Vick Family Foundation for their generous support of this book.

Thank you to the Mayborn conference for the opportunity to participate in a wonderful workshop. Thank you to author Susannah Charleson, who led the workshop, and to my fellow workshop participants for your helpful comments and encouragement. Special thanks to fellow workshop participant Helen Roth for reading my manuscript and making great suggestions.

Special thanks to Sue Friedman for writing the foreword to this book and for founding the wonderful nonprofit organization Facing Our Risk of Cancer Empowered (FORCE). I would have been lost through my decision-making process without the information and support I received from FORCE.

Thank you to Dr. Kelly Hunt, chair and professor, department of breast surgical oncology, division of surgery, at The University of Texas MD Anderson Cancer Center and to Dr. Allison Kurian, associate professor of medicine (oncology) and of health research and policy and director of Women's Clinical Cancer Genetics Program at Stanford University School of Medicine for agreeing to be interviewed for this book and reviewing the accuracy of my references to their research. I am also grateful to CJ Corneliussen-James, founder of METAvivor Research and Support Inc. for her help understanding metastatic breast cancer.

Thank you to my mom, Linda, for sharing your breast cancer story for this book and helping gather family history that documented that even more of our relatives than we initially realized died of what appear to be BRCA2-related cancers.

Thank you to my precious son, Leo, for your patience and support and for putting up with a messy house and perpetual clean laundry shortage as I worked on this project.

I'm eternally grateful for the care I received from genetic counselors, my therapist, breast surgeons, oncologists, nurse practitioners, nurses, hospital techs and other medical professionals, which was excellent and life-saving. Thank you, Bonnie, my dear fellow BRCA2 friend, for hours of listening and talking through difficult decisions and for being there when I had my surgery. And thank you to everyone who encouraged me to write about my experience.

Endnotes

Introduction

1. Angelina Jolie, "My Medical Choice," *The New York Times*, May 14, 2013.

2. Alice Whittemore, et al., "Prevalence of BRCA1 Mutation Carriers among U.S. Non-Hispanic Whites," *Cancer Epidemiology, Biomarkers & Prevention* 13, no. 12 (2004): 2078.

3. National Cancer Institute, "BRCA1 and BRCA2: Cancer Risk and Genetic Testing," website.

4. Timothy R. Rebbeck, et al., "Bilateral Prophylactic Mastectomy Reduces Breast Cancer Risk in BRCA1 and BRCA2 Mutation Carriers: The PROSE Study Group," *Journal of Clinical Oncology* 22 no. 6 (2004): 1055.

5. D. Ford, "Genetic Heterogeneity and Penetrance Analysis of the BRCA1 and BRCA2 Genes in Breast Cancer Families. The Breast Cancer Linkage Consortium," *Am J Hum Genet* 62, no. 3 (1998): 676.

6. Sining Chen and Giovanni Parmigiani, "Meta-Analysis of BRCA1 and BRCA2 Penetrance," *Journal of Clinical Oncology* 25, no. 11 (2007): 1329.

7. Karoline Kuchenbaecker, "Risks of Breast, Ovarian, and Contralateral Breast Cancer for BRCA1 and BRCA2 Mutation Carriers," *JAMA* 317, no. 23 (2017): 2402.

Chapter 1 Welcome to BRCAland

1. *Nature Medicine*, "Lasker Award Winner Mary-Claire King," website.

2. Ford, "Genetic Heterogeneity and Penetrance Analysis," 676.

3. National Cancer Institute, "BRCA1 and BRCA2: Cancer Risk and Genetic Testing," website.

4. Ibid.

5. Ibid.

6. Ibid.

7. Ibid.

8. Ibid.

9. American Cancer Society, "Understanding Your Pathology Report: Atypical Hyperplasia (Breast)," website.

10. National Cancer Institute, "NCI Dictionary of Genetics Terms," website. *https://www.cancer.gov/publications/dictionaries/genetics-dictionary/def/deleterious-mutation*

11. American Cancer Society, "Can Ovarian Cancer Be Found Early?" website.

12. American Cancer Society, "What Are the Key Statistics about Ovarian Cancer?" website.

Chapter 2 Not Simple, Pretty Things

1. Lucas, *Why I Wore Lipstick to My Mastectomy*, 2.

2. American Society of Plastic Surgeons, "2018 Plastic Surgery Statistics," website.

3. Corrie Pikul, "To Cut My Breasts Off or Not to Cut My Breasts Off?" *Salon*, April 2, 2008.

4. *Washington Post*, "Miss D.C. Allyn Rose on her Decision to Opt for a Double Mastectomy after Miss America Pageant."

5. Ibid.

6. Jolie, "My Medical Choice."

7. Liz Neporent, "Angelina Jolie's Mastectomy Fueling National Debate," *ABC News*, June 4, 2013.

8. Maggie Fox and JoNell Aleccia. "More Women Opting for Preventative Mastectomy—But Should They Be?" *NBC News*, May 15, 2013.

9. *NBC News*, "Doctors Approve of Jolie's Surgery," March 24, 2015, website.

10. Joey DiGuglielmo, "Rippin' and Tearin' and Strippin'," *Washington Blade*, June 13, 2013.

11. Ibid.

12. Theodora Ross, *A Cancer in the Family: Take Control of Your Genetic Inheritance* (New York: Avery, 2016), 89.

13. Kelly A. Metcalfe, et al., "International Variation in Rates of Uptake of Preventive Options in BRCA1 and BRCA2 Mutation Carriers." *International Journal of Cancer* 122, no. 9 (2008): 10.

14. Ibid.

15. Ibid.

16. Rebbeck, "Bilateral Prophylactic Mastectomy," 1055.

17. Kelly Hunt, et al., "Society of Surgical Oncology Breast Disease Working Group Statement on Prophylactic (Risk-Reducing) Mastectomy," *Annals of Surgical Oncology* 24, no. 2 (2017): 379.

18. Ibid.

19. Kelly K. Hunt, interview.

20. Facing Our Risk of Cancer Empowered, "Genes Associated with Hereditary Cancer," website.

21. Sunita Desai, et al. "Do Celebrity Endorsements Matter?: Observational Study of BRCA Gene Testing and Mastectomy Rates after Angelina Jolie's *New York Times* Editorial," *BMJ* 355 (2016): 6357.

22. Brian Drohan, et al. "Hereditary Breast and Ovarian Cancer and Other Hereditary Syndromes: Using Technology to Identify Carriers," *Annals of Surgical Oncology* 19 (2012): 1732.

23. Facing Our Risk, "Signs of Hereditary Breast, Ovarian and Related Cancers (HBOC)," website.

24. Claudia Dreifus, "A Never-Ending Genetic Quest: Mary-Claire King's Pioneering Gene Work, From Breast Cancer to Human Rights," *The New York Times*, February 10, 2015.

25. Efrat Gabai-Kapara, et al., "Population-Based Screening for Breast and Ovarian Cancer Risk Due to *BRCA1* and *BRCA2*." *Proceedings of the National Academy of Sciences of the United States of America* 111, no. 39 (2014).

26. Ross, *A Cancer in the Family*, 65.

27. Cynthia Graeber, "Why I Won't Get the Genetic Test for Breast Cancer," *Wired*, September 27, 2016.

Chapter 3 **The Fault in Our Genes**

1. Elaine Schattner, "Chatting with Annie Parker: A Patient's View on How Cancer Care Has Changed Since the 1960s," *Forbes*, March 29, 2015.

2. U.S. Supreme Court Blog, "Association for Molecular Pathology et al v. Myriad Genetics, Inc."

3. Facing Our Risk, "Paying for Genetic Services," website.

4. Karoline Kuchenbaecker, "Risks of Breast, Ovarian, and Contralateral Breast Cancer for BRCA1 and BRCA2 Mutation Carriers," *JAMA* 317, no. 23 (2017): 2402.

5. Ibid.

6. Ibid., 2412.

7. Facing Our Risk, "Understanding BRCA and HBOC Nutrition and Lifestyle," website.

8. Dean Ornish, "For Breast Cancer, It's Not Nature vs. Nurture—It's Both," *Time*, December 18, 2014.

9. Gilda Radner. *It's Always Something* (New York: Simon and Schuster, 1989), 138–139.

Chapter 4 **Pinkwashed**

1. Barbara Ehrenreich, "Welcome to Cancerland: A Mammogram Leads to a Cult of Pink Kitsch," *Harper's Magazine,* November 2001.

2. National Cancer Institute, "Mammograms," website.

3. American Cancer Society, "U.S. Breast Cancer Statistics," website.

4. World Health Organization, "Cancer Fact Sheet: Breast Cancer," website.

5. American Cancer Society, "U.S. Breast Cancer Statistics."

6. Ibid.

7. American Cancer Society, "Understanding a Breast Cancer Diagnosis," website.

8. Joi L. Morris, and Ora K. Gordon, *Positive Results: Making the Best Decisions When You're at High Risk for Breast or Ovarian Cancer* (Amherst, NY: Prometheus Books, 2010), 207.

9. Elizabeth Edwards, *Resilience* (New York: Broadway Books, 2006), 121.

10. Katie Couric, "Elizabeth Edwards Battles Breast Cancer," *NBC News*, November 21, 2004.

11. Cate Edwards, "My Mom's Brave Struggle with Breast Cancer," *CNN Opinion*, October 9, 2013.

12. Joyce O'Shaughnessy, "Extending Survival with Chemotherapy in Metastatic Breast Cancer," *The Oncologist* 10 no. 3, (2005): 20.

13. Carrie Corey, "Living With Stage 4 Breast Cancer: My Semi-Charmed Kind of Life," Cure, accessed September 22, 2018.

14. Laurie Becklund, "As I Lay Dying," *Los Angeles Times,* February 20, 2015.

15. Angela B. Mariotto, et al., "Estimation of the Number of Women Living with Metastatic Breast Cancer in the United States,"*Cancer Epidemiology, Biomarkers & Prevention* 26, no. 6 (2017): 809.

16. Ibid.

17. Ibid.

18. Ibid.

19. Breastcancer.org, "Recurrent Breast Cancer," website.

20. Ehrenreich, "Welcome to Cancerland."

21. Allison Kurian, et al., "Survival Analysis of Cancer Risk Reduction Strategies for BRCA1/2 Mutation Carriers," *Journal of Clinical Oncology* 28, no. 2 (2010): 222.

22. Kurian, interview.

23. Kandice Ludwig, et al., "Risk Reducation and Survival Benefit of Prophylactic Surgery in BRCA Mutation Carriers: A Systematic Review," *The American Journal of Surgery* (2016): 660.

24. Ibid.

Chapter 5 **False Alarms**

1. Andrew Plemmons Pratt, "What to Do with a 'Deleterious Mutation'?" *Science Progress*, July 1, 2008.

2. David Mattos, et al., "Lifetime Costs of Prophylactic Mastectomies and Reconstruction versus Surveillance." *Plastic and Reconstructive Surgery* 136, no. 6 (December 2015): 730e.

3. Helen Blumen, "Comparison of Treatment for Breast Cancer Costs by Stage and Tumor," *American Health and Drug Benefits,* 9, no. 1 (2016): 29.

4. National Cancer Institute, "Many Ovarian Cancers May Start in Fallopian Tubes, Study Finds," website.

5. Facing Our Risk, "Surgical Removal of Ovaries and Tubes," website.

6. Timothy Rebbeck, "Effect of Short-Term Hormone Replacement Therapy on Breast Cancer Risk Reduction After Bilateral Prophylactic Oophorectomy in BRCA1 and BRCA2 Mutation Carriers: The PROSE Study Group," *Journal of Clinical Oncology* 23, no. 31 (2015): 7804.

7. Andrew Kaunitz, "Is Menopausal Hormone Therapy Safe When Your Patient Carries a BRCA Mutation?" *OBG Management* 27, no. 8 (2015): 24.

8. A.P. Finch, et al., "Impact of Oophorectomy on Cancer Incidence and Mortality in Women with a BRCA1 or BRCA2 Mutation." *Journal of Clinical Oncology* 32, no. 15 (2014): 1547.

9. Douglas A. Levine, et al., "Fallopian Tube and Primary Peritoneal Carcinomas Associated With BRCA Mutations." *Journal of Clinical Oncology* 21, no. 22 (2003): 4222.

10. Timothy R. Rebbeck, et al., "Bilateral Prophylactic Mastectomy Reduces Breast Cancer Risk in BRCA1 and BRCA2 Mutation Carriers: The PROSE Study Group," *Journal of Clinical Oncology* 22 no. 6 (2004): 1055.

Chapter 6 The Push

1. Molly Ivins, "Who Needs Breasts Anyway?" *Time*, Feb. 10, 2002.

2. Kelly Hunt, et al., "Society of Surgical Oncology Breast Disease Working Group Statement on Prophylactic (Risk-Reducing) Mastectomy," *Annals of Surgical Oncology* 24, no. 2 (2017): 379.

3. Caroline Helwick, "Nipple-Sparing Surgery Shown to be Safe—And Increasingly Preferred." *The ASCO Post*, September 10, 2016.

4. Amy Colwell, "Breast Reconstruction following Nipple-Sparing Mastectomy: Predictors of Complications, Reconstruction Outcomes, and 5-Year Trends," *Plastic & Reconstructive Surgery* 133, no. 3 (2014): 496.

Chapter 7 **Just Do It**

1. Eleanor Roosevelt, *You Learn by Living* (Westminster: John Knox Press, 2009), 29.

2. Pema Chödrön, *When Things Fall Apart: Heart Advice for Difficult Times* (Boulder, CO: Shambhala Publications, 1986), 157.

3. Sue Friedman, Rebecca Sutphen and Kathy Steligo, *Confronting Hereditary Breast and Ovarian Cancer: Identify Your Risk, Understand Your Options, Change Your Destiny* (Baltimore: Johns Hopkins University Press, 2012), 191.

Chapter 8 **The Angelina**

1. Nora Ephron. "Nora Ephron's Commencement Address to Wellesley Class of 1996," *Huffington Post*, June 26, 2012.

Chapter 9 **Surprise**

1. Judy Blume, "!@#$% Happens." *Judy's Blog*, September 5, 2012.

2. Pink Lotus Breast Center, "A Patient's Journey: Angelina Jolie," website.

3. American Cancer Society, "Ductal Carcinoma in Situ," website.

4. Mayo Clinic, "Ductal Carcinoma in Situ," website.

5. Susan G. Komen, "Ductal Carcinoma in Situ," website.

6. Johns Hopkins Medicine, "Ductal Carcinoma in Situ," website.

Chapter 10 **From A to B**

1. Victoria Dawson Hoff, "Christina Applegate Gets Real about Her Body after Breast Cancer," *Elle*, October 7, 2014.

Chapter 11 **It's Always Something**

1. Radner, *It's Always Something*, 268.

2. Facing Our Risk, "Update on Pancreatic Cancer Genetics Research," website.

3. American Cancer Society, "Pancreatic Cancer Key Statistics," website.

4. Ibid.

5. U.S. Food and Drug Administration, "FDA Evaluating the Risk of Brain Deposits with Repeated Use of Gadolinium-Based Contrast Agents for Magnetic Resonance Imaging (MRI)," website.

6. Radiology Society of North America, "Gadolinium May Remain in Brain after Contrast MRI," website.

7. Facing Our Risk, "Safety of MRI Contrast Agent," website.

8. Denise Grady, "A Shocking Diagnosis: Breast Implants 'Gave Me Cancer,'" *The New York Times*, May 14, 2017.

9. U.S. Food and Drug Administration, "Medical Device Reports of Breast Implant-Associated Anaplastic Large Cell Lymphoma," website.

Bibliography

Books and Articles

Becklund, Laurie. "As I Lay Dying." *Los Angeles Times.* February 20, 2015. *http://www.latimes.com/opinion/op-ed/la-oe-becklund-breast-cancer-komen-20150222-story.html.*

Blumen, Helen, Kathryn Fitch, and Vincent Polkus. "Comparison of Treatment for Breast Cancer Costs by Stage and Tumor." *American Health and Drug Benefits,* 9, no. 1 (2016): 23–32. *https://www.ncbi.nlm.nih.gov/pmc/articles/PMC4822976/*

Borzekowski, Dina L.G., et al. "The Angelina Effect: Immediate Reach, Grasp, and Impact of Going Public." *Genetics in Medicine* 16 (2013): 516–521 *http://www.nature.com/gim/journal/v16/n7/abs/gim2013181a.html?foxtrotcallback=true.*

Campeau, Philippe M., et al. "Hereditary Breast Cancer: New Genetic Developments, New Therapeutic Avenues." *Human Genetics* 124, no. 1 (2008): 31–42. *https://www.ncbi.nlm.nih.gov/pubmed/18575892*

Cook-Deegan, Robert, et al. "After Myriad: Genetic Testing in the Wake of Recent Supreme Court Decisions about Gene Patents." *Current Genetic Medicine Reports* 2, no. 4 (2014): 223–241. *https://www.ncbi.nlm.nih.gov/pmc/articles/PMC4225052/*

Chen, Sining, and Giovanni Parmigiani. "Meta-Analysis of BRCA1 and BRCA2 Penetrance." *Journal of Clinical Oncology* 25, no. 11 (2007): 1329–1333. *https://www.ncbi.nlm.nih.gov/pmc/articles/PMC2267287/*

Chödrön, Pema. *When Things Fall Apart: Heart Advice for Difficult Times.* Boulder, CO: Shambhala Publications Inc., 1986.

Colwell, Amy S. M.D., et al. "Breast Reconstruction Following Nipple-Sparing Mastectomy: Predictors of Complications, Reconstruction Outcomes, and 5-Year Trends." *Plastic & Reconstructive Surgery* 133, no. 3 (2014): 496–506. *https://www.ncbi.nlm.nih.gov/pub med/24572843*

Couric, Katie. "Elizabeth Edwards Battles Breast Cancer." *NBC News.* November 21, 2004. *http://www.nbcnews.com/id/6522712/ns/ dateline_nbc-newsmakers/t/elizabeth-edwards-battles-breast-cancer/#.W6cBZ2hKjIU*

Desai, Sunita, et al. "Do Celebrity Endorsements Matter?: Observational Study of BRCA Gene Testing and Mastectomy Rates after Angelina Jolie's *New York Times* Editorial." *BMJ* 355 (2016): i6357. *https://doi.org/10.1136/bmj.i6357*

DiGuglielmo, Joey. "Rippin' and Tearin' and Strippin'." *Washington Blade.* June 13, 2013. *http://www.washingtonblade.com/2013/ 06/13/rippin-tearin-strippin/*

Domchek, Susan, et al. "Association of Risk-Reducing Surgery in BRCA1 and BRCA2 Mutation Carriers with Cancer Risk and Mortality." *Journal of the American Medical Association (JAMA)* 304, no. 9 (2010): 967–975. *https://www.ncbi.nlm.nih.gov/pmc/ articles/PMC2948529/*

Dreifus, Claudia. "A Never-Ending Genetic Quest: Mary-Claire King's Pioneering Gene Work, From Breast Cancer to Human Rights." *The New York Times.* February 10, 2015. *https://www. nytimes.com/2015/02/10/science/mary-claire-kings-pioneering-gene-work-from-breast-cancer-to-human-rights.html*

Drohan, Brian, et al. "Hereditary Breast and Ovarian Cancer and Other Hereditary Syndromes: Using Technology to Identify Carriers." *Annals of Surgical Oncology* 19 (2012): 1732–1737. *https://www.ncbi.nlm.nih.gov/pubmed/22427173*

Edwards, Cate. "My Mom's Brave Struggle with Breast Cancer." *CNN Opinion.* October 9, 2013. *http://www.cnn.com/2013/10/08/ opinion/edwards-breast-cancer/index.html*

Edwards, Elizabeth. *Resilience.* New York: Broadway Books, 2006.

Ehrenreich, Barbara. "Welcome to Cancerland: A Mammogram Leads to a Cult of Pink Kitsch." *Harper's Magazine.* November 2001. *http://barbaraehrenreich.com/cancerland/*

Ephron, Nora. "Nora Ephron's Commencement Address to Wellesley Class of 1996." *Huffington Post*. June 26, 2012. *<https://www. huffingtonpost.com/2012/06/26/norah-ephrons-commencement-96-address_n_1628832.html>*.

Finch A.P., et al. "Impact of Oophorectomy on Cancer Incidence and Mortality in Women with a BRCA1 or BRCA2 Mutation." *Journal of Clinical Oncology* 32, no. 15 (2014): 1547–1553. *https://www.ncbi.nlm.nih.gov/pubmed/24567435*

Finch, Amy, and Steven A. Narod. "Quality of Life and Health Status after Prophylactic Salpingo-Oophorectomy in Women Who Carry a BRCA Mutation: A Review." *Maturitas: The European Menopause Journal* 70, no. 3 (2011): 261–265. *https://www. ncbi.nlm.nih.gov/pubmed/21893388*

Ford, D., et al. "Genetic Heterogeneity and Penetrance Analysis of the BRCA1 and BRCA2 Genes in Breast Cancer Families. The Breast Cancer Linkage Consortium." *Am J Hum Genet* 62, no. 3 (1998): 676–689. *https://www.ncbi.nlm.nih.gov/pubmed/9497246*

Fox, Maggie, and JoNell Aleccia. "More Women Opting for Preventative Mastectomy—But Should They Be?" *NBC News*. May 15, 2013. *<https://www.nbcnews.com/health/more-women-opting-preventive-mastectomy-should-they-be-1C9918752>*.

Friedman, Sue, Rebecca Sutphen, and Kathy Steligo. *Confronting Hereditary Breast and Ovarian Cancer: Identify Your Risk, Understand Your Options, Change Your Destiny*. Baltimore: The Johns Hopkins University Press, 2012.

Gabai-Kapara, Efrat, et al. "Population-Based Screening for Breast and Ovarian Cancer Risk Due to *BRCA1* and *BRCA2*." *Proceedings of the National Academy of Sciences of the United States of America* 111, no. 39 (2014): 14205–14210. *https:// www.ncbi.nlm.nih.gov/pubmed/25192939*

Grady, Denise. "A Shocking Diagnosis: Breast Implants 'Gave Me Cancer.'" *The New York Times*. May 14, 2017. *https://www. nytimes.com/2017/05/14/health/breast-implants-cancer.html*

Graeber, Cynthia. "Why I Won't Get the Genetic Test for Breast Cancer." *Wired*. September 27, 2016. *https://www.wired.com/ 2016/09/wont-get-genetic-test-breast-cancer/*

Guo, Fangjian. "Use of BRCA Mutation Test in the U.S., 2004–2014." *American Journal of Preventative Medicine* 52, no. 6 (2017): 702–709. *https://www.ncbi.nlm.nih.gov/pubmed/28342662*

Helwick, Caroline. "Nipple-Sparing Surgery Shown to be Safe—And Increasingly Preferred." *The ASCO Post*, September 10, 2016. *http://www.ascopost.com/issues/september-10-2016/nipple-sparing-mastectomy-shown-to-be-safe-and-increasingly-preferred/*

Hoff, Victoria Dawson, "Christina Applegate Gets Real About Her Body After Breast Cancer." *Elle.* October 7, 2014. *http://www.elle.com/culture/celebrities/news/a15024/christina-applegate-breast-cancer-awareness-interview/>.*

Hunt, Kelly, M.D., et al. "Society of Surgical Oncology Breast Disease Working Group Statement on Prophylactic (Risk-Reducing) Mastectomy." *Annals of Surgical Oncology* 24, no. 2 (2017): 375–397. *https://www.ncbi.nlm.nih.gov/pubmed/27933411*

Ivins, Molly. "Who Needs Breasts Anyway?" *Time*, February 10, 2002. *http://content.time.com/time/magazine/article/0,9171,201917,00.html*

Jolie Pitt, Angelina. "Diary of a Surgery." *The New York Times,* March 24, 2015. *https://www.nytimes.com/2015/03/24/opinion/angelina-jolie-pitt-diary-of-a-surgery.html*

Jolie, Angelina. "My Medical Choice." *The New York Times,* May 14, 2013. *https://www.nytimes.com/2013/05/14/opinion/my-medical-choice.html*

Kaunitz, Andrew M. "Is Menopausal Hormone Therapy Safe When Your Patient Carries a BRCA Mutation?" *OBG Management* 27, no. 8 (2015): 24–26.

King, Mary-Claire, et al. "Population-Based Screening for BRCA1 and BRCA2." *JAMA* 312, no. 11 (2014): 1091–1092. *https://jamanetwork.com/journals/jama/fullarticle/1902783*

Kuchenbaecker, Karoline B, et al. "Risks of Breast, Ovarian, and Contralateral Breast Cancer for BRCA1 and BRCA2 Mutation Carriers." *JAMA* 317, no. 23 (2017): 2402–2416. *https://www.ncbi.nlm.nih.gov/pubmed/28632866*

Kurian, Allison W., et al. "Survival Analysis of Cancer Risk Reduction Strategies for BRCA1/2 Mutation Carriers." *Journal of Clinical*

Oncology 28, no. 2 (2010): 222–231. *https://www.ncbi.nlm.nih. gov/pmc/articles/PMC2815712/*

Levine, Douglas A., et al. "Fallopian Tube and Primary Peritoneal Carcinomas Associated With BRCA Mutations." *Journal of Clinical Oncology* 21, no. 22 (2003): 4222–4227. *https://www. ncbi.nlm.nih.gov/pubmed/14615451*

Lucas, Geralyn. *Why I Wore Lipstick to My Mastectomy.* New York: St. Martin's Press, 2004.

Ludwig, Kandice K. M.D., et al. "Risk Reducation and Survival Benefit of Prophylactic Surgery in BRCA Mutation Carriers: A Systematic Review." *The American Journal of Surgery* (2016): 212, 660–669. *https://www.ncbi.nlm.nih.gov/pubmed/27649974*

Mariotto, Angela B., et al. "Estimation of the Number of Women Living with Metastatic Breast Cancer in the United States." *Cancer Epidemiology, Biomarkers & Prevention* 26, no. 6 (2017): 809–815. *http://cebp.aacrjournals.org/content/early/2017/05/05/ 1055-9965.EPI-16-0889*

Mattos, David, et al. "Lifetime Costs of Prophylactic Mastectomies and Reconstruction versus Surveillance." *Plastic and Reconstructive Surgery* 136, no. 6 (December 2015): 730e. *https://journals.lww.com/plasreconsurg/Abstract/2015/12000/ Lifetime_Costs_of_Prophylactic_Mastectomies_and.2.aspx*

Metcalfe, Kelly A., et al. "International Variation in Rates of Uptake of Preventive Options in BRCA1 and BRCA2 Mutation Carriers." *International Journal of Cancer* 122, no. 9 (2008): 2017–2022. *https://www.ncbi.nlm.nih.gov/pmc/articles/PMC2936778/*

Morris, Joi. L., and Ora K. Gordon. *Positive Results: Making the Best Decisions When You're at High Risk for Breast or Ovarian Cancer.* Amherst, NY: Prometheus Books, 2010.

Nature Medicine. "Lasker Award Winner Mary-Claire King, Q&A," 20, no. 10 (October 2014): xxi, accessed September 22, 2018, *http://www.laskerfoundation.org/media/filer_public/e5/45/ e545a94d-f1f2-432d-ad13-944958640657/2014_s_king.pdf.*

NBC News. "Doctors Approve of Jolie's Surgery," March 24, 2015. *https://www.nbcnews.com/health/health-news/doctors-approve- angelina-jolie-s-surgery-n329456*

Neporent, Liz. "Angelina Jolie's Mastectomy Fueling National Debate." *ABC News*, June 4, 2013. *<http://abcnews.go.com/Health/ angelina-jolies-double-mastectomy-fueling-national-debate/ story?id=19315336>*

Ornish, Dean M.D. "For Breast Cancer: It's Not Nature vs. Nurture— It's Both." *Time*, December 18, 2014. *<http://time.com/3640670/ breast-cancer-brca-mutation-lifestyle-genes/>*.

O'Shaughnessy, Joyce. "Extending Survival with Chemotherapy in Metastatic Breast Cancer." *The Oncologist* 10 no. 3, (2005): 20–29.

Pikul, Corrie. "To Cut My Breasts Off, Or Not to Cut My Breasts Off?" *Salon*, April 2, 2008. *<http://www.salon.com/2008/04/02/ jessica_queller/>*.

Plemmons Pratt, Andrew. "What to Do with a 'Deleterious Mutation?'" *Science Progress*, July 1, 2008. *<https://scienceprogress.org/2008/ 07/rudnick-interview/>*.

Queller, Jessica. *Pretty Is What Changes: Impossible Choices, the Breast Cancer Gene, and How I Defied My Destiny*. New York: Spiegel and Grau, 2008.

Radner, Gilda. *It's Always Something*. New York: Simon and Schuster, 1989.

Rebbeck, Timothy R., et al. "Prophylactic Oophorectomy in Carriers of BRCA1 or BRCA2 Mutations." *New England Journal of Medicine* 346, no. 21(2002): 1616–1622.

Rebbeck, Timothy R., et al. "Bilateral Prophylactic Mastectomy Reduces Breast Cancer Risk in BRCA1 and BRCA2 Mutation Carriers: The PROSE Study Group." *Journal of Clinical Oncology* 22 no. 6 (2004): 1055–1062.

Rebbeck, Timothy R., et al. "Effect of Short-Term Hormone Replacement Therapy on Breast Cancer Risk Reduction After Bilateral Prophylactic Oophorectomy in BRCA1 and BRCA2 Mutation Carriers: The PROSE Study Group." *Journal of Clinical Oncology* 23, no. 31 (2015): 7804–7810.

Reddig, A.J., and S. S. McAllister. "Review: Breast Cancer and Metastasis." *Journal of Internal Medicine* 274 no. 2 (2013):113– 126. *https://www.ncbi.nlm.nih.gov/pubmed/23844915*

Roosevelt, Eleanor. *You Learn by Living*. Westminster: John Knox Press, 2009.

Ross, Theodora. *A Cancer in the Family: Take Control of Your Genetic Inheritence*. New York: Avery, 2016.

Schattner, Elaine. "Chatting with Annie Parker: A Patient's View on How Cancer Care Has Changed Since the 1960s." *Forbes*, March 29, 2015. <*https://www.forbes.com/sites/elaineschattner/2015/03/29/chatting-with-annie-parker-a-patients-perspective-on-how-cancer-care-has-changed-since-the-1970s/#fb988561b724*>.

Schwartz, Marc D., et al. "Long-Term Outcomes of BRCA1/BRCA2 Testing: Risk Reduction and Surveillance." *Cancer* 118 no. 2, (2012): 510–17. *https://www.ncbi.nlm.nih.gov/pubmed/21717445*

Washington Post, "Miss D.C. Allyn Rose on her Decision to Opt for a Double Mastectomy after Miss America Pageant," November 19, 2012. *https://live.washingtonpost.com/pb/blogs/reliable-source/post/miss-dc-allyn-rose-on-her-decision-to-opt-for-a-double-mastectomy-after-miss-america-pageant/2012/11/19/b888e7e6-326b-11e2-9cfa-e41bac906cc9_blog.html*

Whittemore, Alice S., et al. "Prevalence of BRCA1 Mutation Carriers among U.S. Non-Hispanic Whites." *Cancer Epidemiology, Biomarkers & Prevention* 13, no. 12 (2004): 2078–83. *https://www.ncbi.nlm.nih.gov/pubmed/15598764*

Websites and Blogs

American Cancer Society, "U.S. Breast Cancer Statistics," accessed September 22, 2018, *https://www.breastcancer.org/symptoms/understand_bc/statistics*.

American Cancer Society, "Can Ovarian Cancer Be Found Early?" accessed September 22, 2018, *https://www.cancer.org/cancer/ovarian-cancer/detection-diagnosis-staging/detection.html*.

American Cancer Society, "Key Statistics for Ovarian Cancer," accessed September 22, 2018, *https://www.cancer.org/cancer/ovarian-cancer/about/key-statistics.html*.

American Cancer Society, "Pancreatic Cancer Key Statistics," accessed September 22, 2018, *https://www.cancer.org/cancer/pancreatic-cancer/about/key-statistics.html*.

American Cancer Society, "Understanding a Breast Cancer Diagnosis," accessed September 22, 2018, *https://www.cancer.org/cancer/ breast-cancer/understanding-a-breast-cancer-diagnosis.html.*

American Cancer Society, "Understanding Your Pathology Report: Atypical Hyperplasia (Breast)," accessed September 22, 2018, *https://www.cancer.org/treatment/understanding-your-diagnosis/ tests/understanding-your-pathology-report/breast-pathology/ atypical-hyperplasia.html.*

American Society of Plastic Surgeons, "2018 Plastic Surgery Statistics," accessed September 22, 2018, *https://www.plasticsur-gery.org/documents/News/Statistics/2017/plastic-surgery-statis-tics-report-2017.pdf.*

Blume, Judy. "!@#$% Happens," Judy's Blog, September 5, 2012, accessed September 22, 2018, *http://judyblumeblog.blogspot.com/ 2012/09/happens.html.*

Breastcancer.org, "Recurrent Breast Cancer," accessed September 22, 2018, *https://www.breastcancer.org/symptoms/diagnosis/recurrent*

Corey, Carrie, "Living With Stage 4 Breast Cancer: My Semi-Charmed Kind of Life," Cure, accessed September 22, 2018, *https://www. curetoday.com/community/carrie-corey?p=2.*

Facing Our Risk of Cancer Empowered, "Breast Cancer Risk in Previvors," accessed September 22, 2018, *http://www.facingour risk.org/understanding-brca-and-hboc/information/risk-factors/ breast-cancer-risks/basics/breast-cancer-risk-in-previvors. php#text.*

Facing Our Risk of Cancer Empowered, "Safety of MRI Contrast Agent," accessed September 22, 2018, *http://www.facingourrisk. org/understanding-brca-and-hboc/information/risk-management/ surveillance-breast-cancer/basics/safety-gadolinium.php*

Facing Our Risk of Cancer Empowered, "Genes Associated with Hereditary Cancer," accessed September 22, 2018, *http://www. facingourrisk.org/understanding-brca-and-hboc/information/ hereditary-cancer/other-genes/.*

Facing Our Risk of Cancer Empowered, "Male Breast Cancer," accessed September 22, 2018, *http://www.facingourrisk.org/ understanding-brca-and-hboc/information/risk-factors/breast-cancer-risks/basics/male-breast-cancer.php#text.*

Facing Our Risk of Cancer Empowered, "Paying for Genetic Services," accessed September 22, 2018 *http://www.facingourrisk.org/understanding-brca-and-hboc/information/finding-health-care/paying_for_testing/basics/insurance_coverage_for_testing.php>*.

Facing Our Risk of Cancer Empowered, "Signs of Hereditary Breast, Ovarian and Related Cancers (HBOC)," accessed September 22, 2018, *http://www.facingourrisk.org/understanding-brca-and-hboc/information/hereditary-cancer/hereditary-genetics/basics/signs-of-hereditary-breast-and-ovarian-cancer.php#text.*

Facing Our Risk of Cancer Empowered, "Surgical Removal of Ovaries and Tubes," accessed July 7, 2018, *http://www.facingourrisk.org/understanding-brca-and-hboc/information/risk-management/oophorectomy/basics/overview.php.*

Facing Our Risk of Cancer Empowered, "Understanding BRCA and HBOC nutrition and lifestlye," accessed September 22, 2018, *http://www.facingourrisk.org/understanding-brca-and-hboc/information/nutrition-lifestyle/diet-nutrition/index.php.*

Facing Our Risk of Cancer Empowered, "Update on Pancreatic Cancer Genetics Research," accessed September 22, 2018, *http://www.facingourrisk.org/get-involved/HBOC-community/BRCA-HBOC-blogs/FORCE/research/update-on-pancreatic-cancer-genetics-research/.*

Johns Hopkins Medicine, "Ductal Carcinoma in Situ (DCIS), accessed September 22, 2018, *https://www.hopkinsmedicine.org/breast_center/breast_cancers_other_conditions/ductal_carcinoma_in_situ.html.*

Susan G. Komen, "Ductal Carcinoma in Situ," accessed September 22, 2018, *https://ww5.komen.org/BreastCancer/DCISIntroduction.html.*

Metastatic Breast Cancer Network, "Incidence and Incidence Rates," accessed September 22, 2018, *http://www.mbcn.org/incidence-and-incidence-rates/.*

Mayo Clinic, "Ductal Carcinoma in Situ (DCIS)," accessed September 22, 2018, *https://www.mayoclinic.org/diseases-conditions/dcis/symptoms-causes/syc-20371889.*

National Cancer Institute, "BRCA Mutations: Cancer Risk and Genetic Testing," accessed September 22, 2018, *https://www.cancer.gov/about-cancer/causes-prevention/genetics/brca-fact-sheet.*

National Cancer Institute, "Mammograms," accessed September 22, 2018, *https://www.cancer.gov/types/breast/mammograms-fact-sheet.*

National Cancer Institute, "Many ovarian cancers may start in fallopian tubes, study finds," National Cancer Institute, November 15, 2017. *https://www.cancer.gov/news-events/cancer-currents-blog/2017/ovarian-cancer-fallopian-tube-origins*

Nature Medicine, "Lasker Award Winner Mary-Claire King," accessed September 22, 2018, *http://www.laskerfoundation. org/media/filer_public/e5/45/e545a94d-f1f2-432d-ad13-944958640657/2014_s_king.pdf.*

Pink Lotus Breast Center, "A Patient's Journey: Angelina Jolie," accessed September 22, 2018, *https://pinklotus.com/powerup/insidethejourney/a-patients-journey-angelina-jolie/.*

Radiology Society of North America, "Gadolinium May Remain in Brain after Contrast MRI," accessed September 22, 2018, *https://press.rsna.org/timssnet/media/pressreleases/14_pr_target. cfm?ID=810.*

Susan G. Komen, "Ductal Carcinoma in Situ," accessed September 22, 2018, *https://ww5.komen.org/BreastCancer/DCISIntroduction. html.*

World Health Organization International Agency for Research on Cancer, "Cancer Fact Sheets: Breast Cancer," accessed September 22, 2018, *https://gco.iarc.fr/today/data/pdf/fact-sheets/cancers/cancer-fact-sheets-15.pdf*

Government Reports

U.S. Food and Drug Administration, "Information on Gadolinium-Based Contrast Agents," accessed September 22, 2018, *https://www.fda.gov/Drugs/DrugSafety/Postmarket DrugSafetyInformationforPatientsandProviders/ucm142882.htm*

U.S. Food and Drug Administration, "Breast Implant-Associated Anaplastic Large Cell Lymphoma (BIA-ACL), accessed September 22, 2018, *https://www.fda.gov/medicaldevices/productsandmedical-procedures/implantsandprosthetics/breastimplants/ucm239995.htm*

U.S. Food and Drug Administration, "Medical Device Reports of Breast Implant Associated Anaplastic Large Cell Lymphoma," accessed

September 22, 2018, *https://www.fda.gov/MedicalDevices/ ProductsandMedicalProcedures/ImplantsandProsthetics/ BreastImplants/ucm481899.htm*

U.S. Food and Drug Administration, "FDA evaluating the risk of brain deposits with repeated use of gadolinium-based contrast agents for magnetic resonance imaging (MRI)," accessed September 22, 2018, *https://www.fda.gov/Drugs/DrugSafety/ ucm455386.htm*.

U.S. Food and Drug Administration, Medical Device Reports of Breast Implant-Associated Anaplastic Large Cell Lymphoma, accessed September 22, 2018, *https://www.fda.gov/MedicalDevices/ ProductsandMedicalProcedures/ImplantsandProsthetics/ BreastImplants/ucm481899.htm*.

U.S. Preventive Services Task Force, "Final Recommendation Statement/ BRCA-related cancer, risk assessment, genetic counseling and genetic testing," accessed September 22, 2018, *https://www.uspreventiveservicestaskforce.org/Page/Document/RecommendationStatementFinal/ brca-related-cancer-risk-assessment-genetic-counseling-and-genetic-testing*.

U.S. Supreme Court, "Association for Molecular Pathology v. Myriad Genetics, Inc.," accessed September 22, 2018, *http:// www.scotusblog.com/case-files/cases/association-for-molecular-pathology-v-myriad-genetics-inc*

Interviews

Corneliussen-James, CJ, founder of METAvivor Research and Support Inc. "Metastatic Breast Cancer," interviewed by Kim Horner, March 2, 2018.

Hunt, Kelly MD, F.A.C.S. Professor and Chair Department of Breast Surgical Oncology, The University of Texas at MD Anderson Cancer Center, Houston Texas, interviewed by Kim Horner, February 6, 2018.

Kurian, Allison W., M.D., M.Sc., Associate Professor of Medicine (Oncology) and of Health Research and Policy, Director, Women's Clinical Cancer Genetics Program, Stanford University School of Medicine, interviewed by Kim Horner, December 4, 2017.